# THE
# COMPLETE
# NEUROTIC

# THE COMPLETE NEUROTIC

## The Anxious Person's Guide to Life

**CHARLES A. MONAGAN**

Illustrations by Mick Stevens

**CHRONICLE BOOKS**
SAN FRANCISCO

ISBN 0-8118-4716-0

Manufactured in the U.S.A.

Designed by Laura Crookston

Distributed in Canada by Raincoast Books
9050 Shaughnessy Street
Vancouver, British Columbia V6P 6E5

Chronicle Books LLC
85 Second Street
San Francisco, California 94105

*I would like to thank the Monagan Foundation
and also the members of my family, who have always
understood that anxiety is just another
word for nothing much to do.*

# CONTENTS

# PREFACE TO THE NEW EDITION

Not much has changed in the realm of neuroses since this book first appeared in 1982. People still avoid stepping on cracks. They wonder excessively when it's safe to go back in the water after eating. They daydream in remarkable detail about winning the lottery but never play it. If anything, we have become more self-absorbed than ever during the past twenty years, floating along together on an ever-rising tide of consumer goods and services aimed expressly at our fears and insecurities. If you had asked me in 1982, I might have been able to see through to today's astonishing growth in the packaging and marketing of breath mints, but I don't think I could have guessed that millions of people would now be dealing with their bad feelings about themselves by injecting botulism into their faces, putting little gurgling fountains on their desks at work, or paying as much as $300 at a spa to have someone place warm stones on their backs while Asian elevator music plinks softly in the background.

The thing is, neurosis is timeless. It is a condition without a cure, but the treatments can be endlessly absorbing and even entertaining. Have you been suffering from anxieties lately? Are you feeling especially vulnerable right now to mad cow disease? Are reports of two possible cases of SARS in a small town in central China making you gulp for air? Have you been beating yourself up because you fell in love with a color for your car that now seems so clearly wrong? Not to worry. We neurotics have figured out ways to cope. We have filled our world with little comforts to help us get through it all, from the simple (brightly wrapped candies, hot tea, white-noise boxes, crossword puzzles, fruit-flavored lip balm) to the rather frighteningly complex and expensive (those companionable little egg-shaped toys from Japan that poop in their "pants" and are afraid of the dark). And now, for the first time in over twenty years, you can add this book to the list of resources that can help you recognize and deal with (or repress) your neurotic traits.

This reissuing of what was originally called *The Neurotic's Handbook* adds an additional chapter from my book *The Reluctant Naturalist,* makes a few small revisions to dates, and quietly excises a chapter on the "world view" dealing with the Soviet Union and Warsaw Pact countries. Other than that, all remains as it was first written. Some of the references may seem nostalgic to older readers (ah, those were the days) or incomprehensible to younger readers (ah, the splendor of youth). The headlines may change from day to day, but the human condition emphatically does not. We are as jumpy today as we were when saber-toothed tigers were nosing around just beyond the light of the cooking fire. We need reassurance that we aren't alone and that a twitching muscle in your eyelid doesn't (necessarily) mean you are about to have a stroke. I'm very happy and proud that *The Complete Neurotic* can once again serve that noble cause.

—C.A.M.

# INTRODUCTION

It was not so long ago that most people were normal. They tilled the fields or worked hard in factories, they ate regular food that was hot and plentiful and served on thick crockery, they went to sleep shortly after it got dark, they prayed (all the time, not just when they were in trouble), and they engaged in sex under the covers with the lights out.

Other things in life were normal, too. Buildings had windows that opened and closed and features such as cornices that were pleasing to the eye. Paintings were of people or pleasant land-scapes or boats or bowls of fruit, and patrons bought these paintings at reasonable prices and hung them in their homes and felt happy and at ease living with them. Children were given names such as Joe or Ed or Ann rather than obscure crossword-puzzle names from the Bible or multisyllabic joke names that once would have been reserved for the family dinghy or a pet turtle. There were exceptions to all of this, of course, but for the most part normalcy prevailed and the people were glad just to be alive.

Back then, people
looked like this:

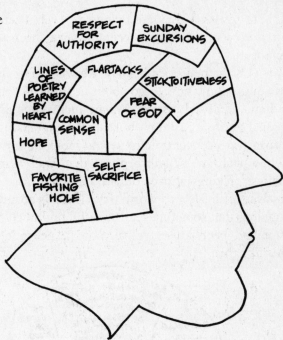

Today, on the other hand, almost no one is normal. If you ask people today whether or not they are "content with their lot" (a key phrase from the lost Age of Normalcy), they will assume that you are talking about real estate and tell you they are not. Unbidden, they will then go on to tell you that they have taken up a terrific new physical activity (and describe in great detail an injury to prove it), that they just bought a new car but wish they'd gotten a different color, that they wished they were single again (if married) or married (if not), that their privet hedge is proving to be much too much of a responsibility, that they are bored at work, overweight but dieting, tempted to enter into a dangerous love affair. They would like to move, maybe far away.

They are restless. They are dying to travel. There are no good men around anymore, no decent women, no leaders, no juicy tomatoes.

This is the neurotic's heyday. We wish to be fulfilled but we don't quite know how to go about it, so we become overstimulated and confused instead. We are lucky enough to have great personal freedom just now, but rather than making us truly free, it drives us to concentrate more and more on ourselves until we reach a state of self-absorption that was once the special province of kings and cardinals. Like them, we begin to take ourselves seriously in a world that clearly is absurd. This causes difficulties that sometimes are dreadful but much more often are minor and peculiar. A typical modern neurotic, for instance, looks like this:

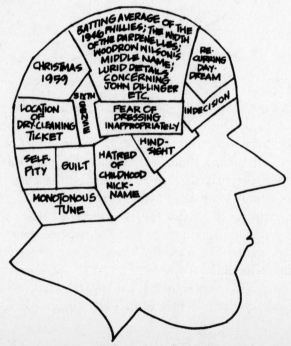

For some time it has been said that you *have* to be neurotic just to get along in the modern world. This is not true, of course, but it has the ring of truth and it is comforting to those of us who frantically change our clothes three times before leaving for a party or who are secretly addicted to grape-flavored lip balm or who believe that losing a finger is preferable to missing the beginning of a movie.

This book doesn't assume that everyone *has* to be neurotic, but it believes that they are anyway. The book is meant to be both a guide and a comfort. It will tell you what to do when you are caught in certain neurotic circumstances, and it should reassure you that what you do in certain other circumstances is not so very odd after all. There is sex here (or what passes for sex), there is hot weather and cold, there is a list of famous neurotics and a few slams against the French. The wonders of baking soda are discussed, as are Ace bandages, palm readings, blind dates, and the fear that someday you'll cross your eyes and they'll *stay* crossed.

This book deals with the real world. It is concerned with the countless petty problems and anxieties that race through your head from the moment you wake up in the morning to the time you go to sleep at night. The main idea here is that we're all in this thing together; we all have trouble getting through the day from time to time. The book will help. If you just pick it up and read it, for example, there's two or three hours killed right there.

# LIFE ITSELF

The Seven Ages of the Neurotic

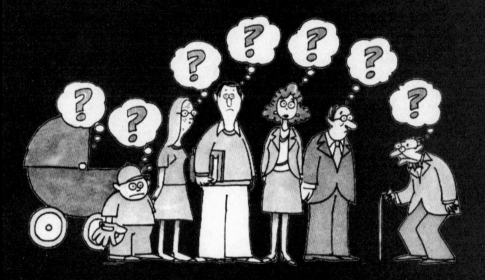

# THE INFANT NEUROTIC

It all begins with pleasing warmth and comfort, with the purr of soft, indistinct voices, and with the soothing ebb and flow of water running nearby. It is the womb, and we'll never have things quite so good again.

Because the world and all its unpleasantness can never live up to the promise of those first nine months, the sheer excellence of the womb can be blamed for almost all future neurotic complaints. Indeed, many neurotics spend a great deal of time trying to approximate the ambience of the womb in later life. They hang around in laundromats, they become wistful and drowsy on dark autumn afternoons when a steady rain is beating against the roof and windows, they find unaccountable pleasure in the droning of a fan or dishwasher. Exceptional neurotics will go so far as to lurk quietly in dark closets (praying that they don't get caught) or build houses near murmuring brooks. They would agree that the womb is wasted on the very, very young.

It is not long before the extraordinary peace and perfection of life is shattered, however. Following the unasked-for trauma of birth itself, the storm clouds begin to gather as soon as someone hangs a frightening, ominously bobbing mobile over the

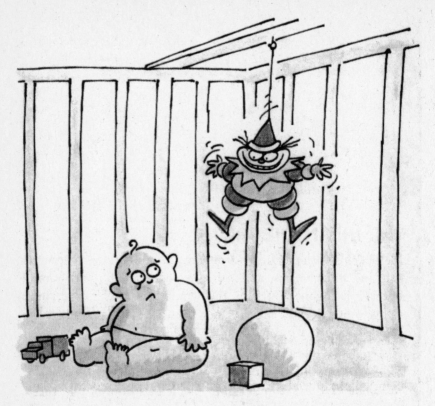

crib. This unsettling (and unavoidable) intrusion usually is accompanied by a parade of adults, each of whom insists upon leaving an impression that is supposed to be memorable but that more often is just puzzling (the fish face; strange trilling noises; mock scoldings). Like a succession of charmless acts in a night-marish vaudeville show, the difficulties of life begin to reveal themselves. From here it is a mere toddle on to the fundamental building blocks of anxiety: distrust, fantasy, insecurity, persecution, and guilt.

1. **DISTRUST.** The pacifier is the first of the many great hoaxes that life holds in store for us. No sooner have we settled into the wonders of the mothering breast than we are tricked into accepting the scant fruit of this cheap, toylike substitute. Is there anything more pitifully defenseless than the wide-eyed babe who is sucking hopefully on a pacifier? Is there ever again any reason for the child to trust anyone once this con game has been found out?

2. **FANTASY.** It is hard to make friends with people who are six times bigger than you are and who very rarely have anything to say that makes any sense. It is much better to have a stuffed animal that you can boss around. The stuffed animal's job is to let the human call all the shots, to offer any necessary solace, to drink imaginary liquids, and to be discarded and resurrected on a nearly daily basis. All of this the animal does without question, thus assuring the child's dissatisfaction with real people and encouraging perpetual flights of fancy.

3. **INSECURITY.** Although it doesn't seem so to the parents, infants are left alone quite a bit of the time. During this leisure time they mainly fret and wonder if anyone ever is coming back to see them again—feelings that neurotics carry with them well into adulthood. Usually, the last thing a parent does before departing is to cover the infant with its blanket: thus the link between blanket and parent, and thus the "security blanket." The blanket offers an illusion of security that in the end is counterproductive and anxiety-producing. The blanket is later given up in favor of gin.

4. **PERSECUTION.** The infant, knowing nothing, wishes to learn something of its world. It wishes to see, to touch, to put in its mouth. For such fledgling efforts at self-education it is thrown into jail, euphemistically known as a playpen. The

playpen is not a rehabilitative facility; the word is a short-ened form of *playpenitentiary,* and it is meant to teach us early on that too much fun is a bad thing and that there always is someone who knows better than we do.

5. **GUILT.** Toilet training introduces us to guilt. This sudden and unseemly preoccupation with our own effluence catches us by surprise, as do the scoldings that come when we are dis-covered with our diapers full. We know that we are doing something wrong, but we can't seem to help it. We feel guilty. Soon we will become more sophisticated, and we will learn to feel guilty even when we do things that are right.

# THE CHILD NEUROTIC

Our formal introduction to anxiety and attendant neurotic behavior comes at the exact moment when we first hear: "Step on a crack, break your mother's back." These words have an immediate and profound effect on the way we look at things (not to mention the way we walk). We perceive for the first time that harmony and happiness hang in the most delicate balance and that unless we are forever vigilant the world easily can dissolve into chaos. We are almost positive that the words them-selves can't be true, yet we take them to heart. After all, who wants to be the one child in a million who knowingly steps on a crack only to come home and find his or her mother writhing in pain on the living room floor?

Anxiety assaults neurotic children from other directions as well. For a while they are allowed to drift happily in a genderless limbo, but once gender identification begins it is as relentless as it is confusing. Little boys must not wear white ice skates. Little girls must not spit hawkers. Little boys do not practice dancing with each other. Little girls do not goose each other on the playground. Gradually, the world turns out to be a place of rules and conformity. Sometimes the rules are simple (don't wear sneakers on the escalator) and sometimes they are difficult (do be a responsible child, but no one likes a tattletale). Always the rules are meant to be obeyed.

Because neurotic children are nothing if not resourceful, they have many ways of battling the pressure to conform. The first of these is to become convinced that they were adopted. If this were true, it would explain so much—the curse of alienation, particularly evident in "family" snapshots; the steady flow of perfunctory birthday presents; the extreme dislike for brussels sprouts while everyone else in the family eats them with great pleasure. Any questions regarding adoption are met with hollow reassurances and even forged documents until the child, with great force of will, decides to make the best of an obviously fishy situation and live on as if everything were aces.

Imaginary friends are another aid to the child who has trouble dealing with the cryptic ways of the world. These friends fall into the scheme of things somewhere between stuffed animals and gin, and they can be of any gender or age, although usually they are contemporaries of the same sex as the child. Imaginary friends lead volatile lives. They are shipwrecked, hit by cars, fall off roofs, come down with the measles. They spill things, break things, stay out late, and don't go to church. They are later replaced by *real* imaginary friends.

The most common way for the child neurotic to break away from the rapidly conforming crowd is to come up with a distinctive physical complaint. This is a trait that becomes much more finely developed in later life, but it can have rather interesting beginnings as well. An important early discovery is Band-Aids. These plastic bandages (available in a splendid array of colors and shapes) can be placed on any sort of cut or scratch, thus calling attention to it and granting it legitimacy. The child is quick to learn that people want to know what is under the Band-Aid and how it got there, and that they will believe just about anything.

Stitches are even better. Stitches bespeak a life that is at least slightly reckless and nonconformist and therefore desirable. The more stitches, the better.

Casts and crutches (assuming they are temporary) are excellent attention-grabbers, too, as are the embellished tales that inevitably go along with them. Particularly anxious children will have every square inch of their casts filled with signatures and Magic Marker doodles (including at least one daisy or Maltese cross), even if they have to do most of the drawing themselves.

A tonsillectomy is perhaps the medical nirvana for the child neurotic. It is a minor procedure, yet not without the possibility of dire consequences. The welfare of the child for a week or so becomes the sole concern of family and friends. The inability to speak for a while after the operation is not only weird and thrilling, but it also greatly increases the solicitude of those who come to visit. Finally, the hospital identification tag is something that you can keep and put on again whenever you need it.

## THE TEENAGE NEUROTIC

Although puberty as a physical process takes only a few years to blaze its hirsute trail, its consequences reverberate like a cannon shot down through all the teenage years. The coming of age is a disruptive shock to both body and mind, and it sends showers of sparks in directions that are unpredictable to say the least. Neurosis is the natural state for teenagers to be in, and it doesn't take much scouting around to see why:

1.  ***The whole world is against teenagers.*** Although many neurotics believe this to be true for all their lives, it is actually true only when they are in their teens. In the eyes of their elders, teens are either overgrown children or childish adults and only time can straighten them out. Adults in places as diverse as Belgium, Peru, and New Zealand agree.

2.  ***Teenagers' parents are strange and intractable.*** Up until this point, Mom and Dad haven't been too bad—a few unnecessarily stern warnings here, a few social gaffes there, but generally okay. Now all of a sudden they seem determined to make up for lost time. Just about everything they say and do is a hideous embarrassment. They can't be trusted in public places. They can't be introduced to your friends without making some ridiculous comment. They insist on advancing ideas that are shopworn and without merit. They think they own you.

3.  ***Teenagers begin to experience powerful yearnings that can no longer be satisfied by Saturday-morning cartoons on TV.*** The problem here is that the teenager's body has landed in a strange new territory before the brain has learned to speak the language. At first these yearnings are so indistinct that girls mistakenly take up horseback riding, while boys go for football and fast cars.

4.  ***With only algebra, English composition, and maybe a little French or Spanish to guide them, teenagers suddenly have to decide how to dress, how to look, how to act, and what to say.*** So they take the only sane course under the circumstances: They wear identical clothes, they strive to achieve the same "look," they all act the same, and they all say the same things.

5.  *Teenagers have nothing to do.* Unless you consider dancing in front of the mirror, doing each other's hair, volunteering for a menial job at the state hospital, or caddying fun things to do. Much better to hang out in a parking lot, smashing bottles and smirking at passersby.

6.  *Teenagers have heard that acne goes away eventually, but they believe that an exception can and will be made in their case.* They also firmly believe that the more important the social occasion, the greater the likelihood that a pimple the size and intensity of an automobile's taillight will appear to cast its unrosy glow over the proceedings.

## THE COLLEGIATE NEUROTIC

The youthful neurotic's personality continues to wobble uncertainly during the college years, but the focus of anxiety gradually shifts over to the question of what he or she will *do* after graduation day. This question invites three basic approaches:

1.  The most extreme neurotics have their whole lives mapped out on a piece of paper that they frequently pull out of a desk drawer and stare at. These people have known what they wanted to be ever since they saved a bird with a broken wing when they were eight years old, and heaven help anyone or anything that gets in their way. Such students do not partake in dormitory hijinks, they wear pajamas to bed, and they believe that the best way to start the day is with a good breakfast. They can be spotted walking across campus engaging various professors in animated conversation or rushing back to the dorm after an exam to look up the answers. Their rooms are very tidy. Their stereo equipment is below par. They often have a few pieces of fruit on the

windowsill. They already know how many children they want to have, and when, and what their names will be.

If these students are nudged even for a moment from their designated path, they easily can fall into a wild tailspin that ends up with them sleeping in the Bowery or wandering through India with no shoes on. They should be joshed good-naturedly but not asked pointed questions about the meaning of life.

2. The second group of collegiate neurotics comprises those who go through a half-dozen or so complete personality changes in the course of the four years. These are the students who are so undecided about themselves and their futures that they react to college society as if it were a succession of masquerade parties, and to the curriculum as if it were a penny candy display. It seems merely a matter of luck and timing as to whether they leave school as future brain surgeons, tree surgeons, or Moonies.

   These people embrace each new thing (a particular brand of beer, a dance step, sociology) with initial enthusiasm and eventual disillusionment. They try on majors as others might try on shoes: looking for something that fits and is practical yet stylish. They do not wish to make any decision regarding the future because if it turns out to be the wrong one, they will have no one to blame but themselves. They hope that if they try enough approaches, the correct course of life will become obvious. It never becomes obvious.

3. The last group of neurotic collegians practices avoidance behavior. They avoid going to classes, avoid establishing even so much as eye contact with professors, avoid joining campus activities, and avoid wearing the school colors to football games. Instead, they ingest great quantities of mind-altering

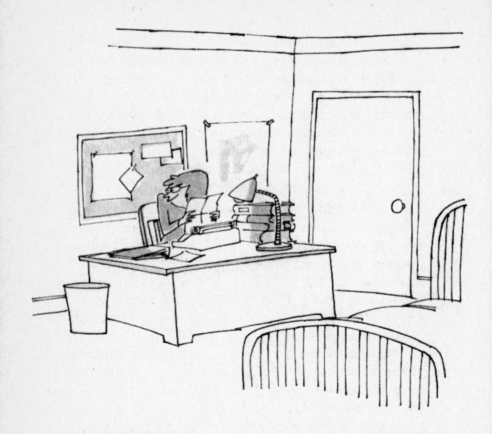

substances and stay in their rooms listening to rock music. They believe that the answers to life lie in rock music rather than in the consequences of the Battle of Tours or in the uses of light and shadow in *The Scarlet Letter*. Because this assumption cannot be proven wrong, these students often are kicked out of school by insecure administrators.

Other forms of typical collegiate avoidance behavior include epic sleeping jags ("I think I have mono"), reversions to childlike behavior ("Hello, Daddy? I don't like it here anymore"), unrequited love ("My whole life is ruined"), and political activism ("Your whole life is ruined").

If any of these students manage to make their way through the full term at college, it probably is only because they felt guilty enough to rouse themselves for a series of all-nighters. The all-nighter is a neurotic exercise that combines a Kafkaesque despair with the tension of the Cuban Missile Crisis. Things learned during an all-nighter are remembered for ten hours, tops, and then forgotten for all time (even under torture or hypnosis).

# THE YOUNG ADULT NEUROTIC

Much has always been made in this country of one's thirtieth birthday. It used to be said that if a man had not found a proper niche in society by age thirty, he was likely to be a shiftless ne'er-do-well and a bounder, and that if a woman had not found a husband by that time, she was doomed to spinsterhood in the most chilling, Agnes Moorehead sort of way. Now, it seems, such opinions are not so widely aired. Neurotics know, however, that people secretly still believe them to be true.

This societal duplicity makes things confusing for young adults. Should they seek independence, they wonder, which is held before them as the mighty beacon of happiness? Or should they seek responsibility, which stands as the only road to fulfillment? By age thirty, most neurotics can be spotted with one foot on the beacon and one on the road. This is not only uncomfortable and ungainly, but it also casts a scary shadow.

Such is the confusion these days that only three things can be said to be completely true regarding the thirtieth birthday.

1. If you haven't got things figured out by now, you never will. You once thought that getting your driver's license would reveal the key to life. Then you thought that going away to school or living out on your own and having your own plants to water would solve things. By age thirty you can see that the answers do not come quite so easily. If you still can't open a bag of potato chips without using your teeth, how are you going to pick apart the subtleties of the cosmos?

2. People who are thirty act as if they are eighteen or forty-six, but they never act as if they are thirty. There is no such thing as acting as if you are thirty.

3. What you knew at age six is much more important than anything you have learned since. You knew pain, fear, anger, envy, love, food, and sleep when you were six. On the other hand, when was the last time you heard someone mention the Huguenots or Planck's constant except in a mildly humorous light? When were you last asked to parse a sentence?

Fortunately, most young adults—particularly those who are just past thirty—begin to try to bury their anxieties behind a facade of normality. They like to be observed as having things well in hand, and they are much more likely to talk calmly about firewood or traffic conditions than they are to rant on and on about someone at work who keeps stealing their paper clips. It is not important that the content of those quiet chats about firewood and traffic is completely neurotic. What is important is that the tone of voice has softened and that outwardly neurotic buzz-words such as *humungous* and *gross* and *teeny-weeny* have been dropped. Life becomes a matter of reserve and grim acceptance, except among the very closest of friends.

# THE MIDDLE-AGED NEUROTIC

The midlife crisis is something that catches everyone but neurotics by surprise. Neurotics expect a crisis at midlife because they have had one at every other age and by now there is reason to believe that only death can stop them. Because they are so practiced at facing crises, neurotics have ready answers for all the deep and desperate questions that arise at this stage of the game. They may not be the *correct* answers, but with questions like these, what difference does it make?

*Who am I?* I am the same person as always, only now with graying hair and a heart that could give out at any moment.

*Where am I?* In the living room, sitting in front of the television but holding the afternoon newspaper up in front of my face so that it looks like I'm not just wasting time.

*What am I doing here?* I am listening to the television. The guest host is just now revealing the exact date of his forthcoming appearance in Las Vegas.

*No, I mean what am I doing here on Earth?* Frankly, I wish I knew. I had a pretty good grasp on it just the other night in a dream, but I couldn't remember the dream when I woke up in the morning. I just remembered the feeling of having a grasp and that it was surprisingly uncomplicated. One thing I *can* do exceptionally well is drive a car in reverse just by looking through the rearview mirror, although I wouldn't claim that as a calling or a reason for living or anything like that.

*What are these things?* These are what are known as possessions. The chair here allows me to sit up or to lounge, according to my whim. The couch unfolds into a bed that is more comfortable than any other in the house. On the wall are framed scenes of idealized family life. The ball is for the dog. There are many other things, all paid for, all insured.

*What is this in my hand?* A martini.

*Who are these people?* They are my family, three children and one mate. They give me a feeling of substance and meaning, I suppose. The children are old enough to be developing distinct neurotic personalities of their own now. Their cuteness has completely disappeared, and they have rejected every bit of advice that I have ever tried to give them.

*What is important?* The martini. The extra olive. The feel of the cold glass against my fingers.

*What else?* Flowers, puppies, balloons, walks in the park, things like that.

*What is unimportant?* Promotions at work, what other people think of me, our daughter's arrest record, the neighbor's dog that shits all over the front lawn.

*What lies beyond life, beyond death?* Hey, what *is* this, some kind of *inquisition?* "What lies beyond life, beyond death?" What the hell is *that* supposed to mean? Why don't you go ask Carl Sagan? Leave me out of it. Leave me alone.

## THE AGED NEUROTIC

The neurotic can be said to have reached old age as soon as he or she becomes considered an eccentric and his or her persistent ranting and raving are fondly classified as irascibility. The key to neurotic behavior in old age is that the ranting is more and more focused on concerns that younger people consider to be unimportant and even petty, such as the welfare of pigeons and the snappish attitude of the newspaper boy.

It is a well-documented phenomenon that the old begin to act like the very young, and this certainly is true of neurotics. The carefully constructed reserve and self-denial of middle age gradually peel away, exposing once again the fundamental core of vulnerability and anxiety that last characterized late childhood (but that always has been bubbling just under the surface). Aged neurotics once again dress just the way they want. Once they realize that they can get away with it, they again refuse to eat certain vegetables. They finally feel free to say whatever they damn well please.

In old age we return to the basic building blocks of anxiety that once shaped our infant lives: distrust, fantasy, insecurity, persecution, and guilt. The specifics of each of these may be different, but the feelings are exactly the same as they always have been: unpleasant.

1.  **DISTRUST.** The distrust that began with the pacifier and then moved on to include baby-sitters, teachers, guidance counselors, so-called friends, plumbers, employers, offspring, and spouses comes to rest finally with doctors. The doctors don't tell you anything or, if they do, they lie. They think you want things made easy for you, but if they took a little time to get to know you, they'd realize you're not like that. The only people the doctors level with are your children, who have begun to visit more often and treat you with affection after years of nothing but abuse. For that to happen, you must be dying. Six months to live, or even less. The doctors (all four or five of them) continue to smile and say everything is fine. The only one you really *can* trust is the chiropractor, but everyone just smiles in a strange way whenever you mention him.

2. **FANTASY.**

   "They don't make 'em like they used to."

   "Dempsey would've cleaned the floor with these guys."

   "We were young and didn't have a care in the world."

   "Nobody could beat your grandmother's cooking."

   "The winters were colder then, and it snowed and snowed and snowed."

   "The city streets were clean and safe."

   "We had to walk four miles to school."

   "Nobody could hit like Hornsby."

   "Those were the days."

3. **INSECURITY.** The paperboy is on drugs. The bus driver's brother-in-law is mixed up with the Mafia. The police spend all their time eating donuts and drinking coffee. The young woman who moved in across the street has visitors at all hours. The reason the Social Security check is for more money now is that they were cheating me before. The Bingo is fixed. The city keeps giving me the runaround about the broken streetlight out front. The mailman didn't tell me he was going on vacation. They moved Merv Griffin to a different channel and now I can't find him. The paperboy is on drugs. The bus driver's brother-in-law is mixed up with the Mafia. The police spend all their time . . .

4. **PERSECUTION.** If the aged neurotic becomes uninhibited enough that he or she begins having too much fun, there exists the threat of being tossed into the slammer, euphemistically known as a rest home. In the rest home, the neurotic is surrounded by people who *really* belong there, and he or she is the one who is politely referred to as a "cau-

tion" by the other residents. The rest home is the ultimate extension of the infant's playpen, and it teaches us for the very last time that having too much fun is a bad thing and that there always is someone who knows better than we do.

5.  **GUILT.** In the end there is no such thing as guilt, because either the Lord is all-forgiving or there is no Lord.

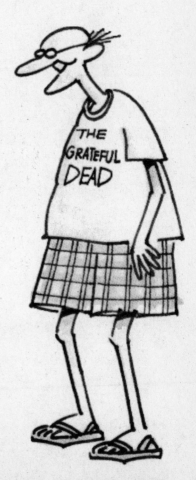

# INSIDE ANXIETY

## The Private Lives of Neurotics

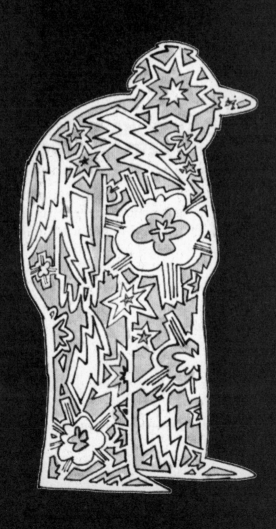

## FIFTEEN OBSERVATIONS REGARDING THE SOCIAL AND PERSONAL BEHAVIOR OF NEUROTICS

1. Neurotics place an unseemly emphasis on being on time. They will leave the house much earlier than is necessary (after being dressed and ready to go for up to three hours) in order to get to their destination. They then will drive around the block or just sit in the car, listening to the radio, until several other guests are seen to arrive and go inside.

2. Neurotics hate to ask directions. This is particularly true of males, who like to think of themselves as self-sufficient trail-blazers even if they are just trying to get to a cocktail party across town.

3. Neurotics daydream about winning the lottery, but they never play it.

4. Neurotics write contentious comments in the margins of books.

5. If there is one chance in a million of making a mistake, a neurotic will not call another person by name.

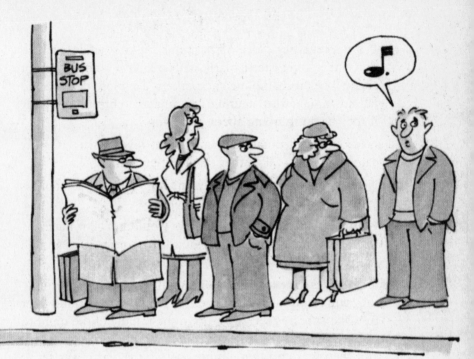

6. Neurotics have favorite coffee cups that they love beyond reason. Exceptional neurotics will go so far as to take these cups with them when they go out for breakfast.

7. Neurotics make a very big deal out of things like *Peter and the Wolf* and *The Wizard of Oz*.

8. Neurotics believe in bumper-sticker wisdom. A car that is covered with bumper stickers has a driver behind the wheel whose mind probably is not on the road.

9. The record collections of neurotics are in alphabetical order. No unauthorized hand is allowed to touch these records. No unauthorized dust is allowed to collect on them.

10. Neurotics hum or whistle at inappropriate times and places.

11. If a neurotic begins to think about walking while walking down the street (particularly with people watching), he or she will begin shambling and perhaps even lose balance and fall down. Likewise, neurotics are unable to breathe properly if they begin thinking about breathing.

12. Neurotics tend to take up causes that involve whales, stray cats, and baby seals rather than human beings.

13. Neurotics are sure the phone will begin ringing as soon as they get out of earshot.

14. Neurotics see omens where others would not. For instance: If the next man who walks around the corner is wearing a hat, it will mean that I can afford to buy the green dress.

15. If neurotics have to get up particularly early in the morning, they will set the alarm clock, check it again ten minutes later to make sure it is set, wake up in the middle of the night to check it again (and make sure the electricity hasn't gone off), and then wake up two minutes before the alarm was set to ring anyway.

## FROM THE MAILBAG

In every town and city in this nation there are certain neurotics who believe it is part of their civic duty to write letters to the editor every four or five days. The names of these people, if not their faces, are familiar to anyone who regularly reads the local newspaper. The letters themselves are longish and often rife with intimations of persecution and conspiracy. Sometimes the writers are experts in one field (fluoridation; highway safety) and feel obliged to hammer home the same point over and over again. More often, however, these correspondents are scholars in all subjects, able to handle local sewer politics and sensitive global affairs with equal aplomb.

Here are excerpts from letters written by five major neurotic types:

## The Watchdog

"Why is the city destroying all its shade trees? Am I the only one to notice that there seems to be an organized program—orchestrated from the mayor's office—to cut down every elm, oak, and maple tree on city property? Maybe I'm just seeing things, but I believe the time has come for the plain people to band together and do something before it's too late. . . . Where will it all end? Will the people next have to guard the trees on their *own* property from the exalted, loot-hungry gang in City Hall? The citizens demand and deserve an answer. Come on, Mister Mayor! We are waiting!"

## The Moralist

"For years I have been living under the misapprehension that yours was a family newspaper, fit for consumption by young and old alike. Now the scales have been taken away from my eyes. If my teenagers wish to learn about venereal disease (which they don't, I can assure you), our family doctor is very well qualified to tell them. . . . Aren't we already surrounded by enough trash without having more delivered to our front door every day?"

## The Hard-Liner

"The electric chair is too good for these animals . . . see them squirm . . . dungeons not such a bad idea . . . punks . . . sticks in my craw . . . two-by-four . . . scum . . . back where they came from . . . soap."

## The Language Snob

"I am quite taken by your quaint but moronic use of 'from whence' in your lead editorial of Tuesday last. Had you bothered to do your homework in fifth grade, you would have learned that such a juxtaposition constitutes a tautology at best and a pleonasm at worst. Please do try to refrain from such bracing excursions into the otiose, or, better yet, go back to a less intellectually taxing pursuit, such as writing paid obituary notices."

## The Animal Lover

"I have a comment for the person who recently wrote the letter that stated, 'The electric chair is too good for these animals.' I would just like to ask that person what kind of animals he is talking about. Squirrels? Rabbits? Does? Little spaniel puppies? Animals don't carry guns or knives. They don't mug you and then kill you because you only had two dollars. Animals live in peace in this world. I'd like to see that writer get *his* head caught in a bear trap and ask him what he thinks then."

# BIZARRE INFLUENCES

There is something in the nature of the neurotic that loves things such as horoscopes and palm readings and the like. Part of this fascination has to do with the neurotic's self-absorption, to be sure, but part also is due to the convenient idea that our fates may not be entirely under our own control. We are perfectly willing to accept any good fortune that comes along as a product of our own design, but it is handy to be able to blame bad luck on some grand and sinister force.

The thing is, it's hard to tell which astrologer or which palm reader to believe. You pick up three daily papers and you get three different horoscopes, each one vaguer than the last. You wonder where the "unexpected journey" will take you and which "coworker" will need your "advice." Similarly, when someone who is trying to pick you up in a bar reads your palm, you don't know whether to laugh or cry or call a cab.

What follows should clear up your doubts once and for all.

## Your Horoscope for the Rest of Your Life

**ARIES** *(March 21–April 19):* Your worst suspicions always will be confirmed. You develop an overpowering taste for veal in late 2007, and this causes confusion at home during the holidays. Romance beckons often, but it disappears whenever you leave the room to put things from the washer into the dryer. You meet and have lunch with a dead ringer for Rudyard Kipling in 2014. Your book, *How to Make Small Talk,* rushes to the top of the best-seller lists and assures your financial security.

**TAURUS** *(April 20–May 20):* You will continue to forget where you hid things. A practical joke you try to pull in August 2010 back-fires and you are forced to run home without any clothes on. Late in your career, coworkers admit you are worth more than they are, and they go on strike until you are given a substantial raise. Hold on to the car you now own—one day it will be declared a classic and fetch an enormous sum of money. Don't automatically ignore those Falling Rock Zone signs just because everybody else does.

**GEMINI** *(May 21–June 21):* The spiritual meanderings never really do stop. You are haunted by the delivery, in January 2015, of a crate of oranges and grapefruit from Florida with only the word *Thanks* on the gift card. Keep away from strangers with beards during the Labor Day weekend of 2009. You are asked several times to appear on television commercials, but you turn down each offer (and all the cash that goes with them) because you really don't believe in the products. Stay away from the Bengal tiger cage at the zoo.

**CANCER** *(June 22–July 22):* A life of gathering useless information. In February 2012, you accidentally wear someone else's raincoat home from a party and, although you always mean to, you never return it. A strange but harmless disease brings you notoriety.

You learn some good card tricks while on vacation in April 2028. Again and again you fall in love with people who are too good for you, but you never learn your lesson.

**LEO** *(July 23–August 22):* No end in sight for restless self-appraisal. In 2010 and again in 2013 you help major celebrities out of embarrassing situations and keep your promises never to tell anyone. Be careful while fooling around with a fuse box in 2024. A love interest flees with the silverware but otherwise leaves behind pleasant memories. Obey all signs in 2011, particularly the one that says, "Do not stand up in the rollercoaster car."

**VIRGO** *(August 23–September 22):* A life of impossible choices. On July 16, 2019, you hear a joke that's so good you can never again recall it without laughing aloud. In 2015 you look directly into a solar eclipse with no ill effects whatsoever. After spending a short period of time in a sensory deprivation chamber, you begin demanding a linen napkin at every meal. In late 2011 you and your pet are invited to appear on *The Tonight Show*.

**LIBRA** *(September 23–October 23):* Continued specious self-improvement. In 2020 an undetected head injury sustained in a minor automobile accident causes you to overtip extravagantly. If you accept an invitation to dine with a man wearing a jewel-encrusted fez, you get what you deserve. On an unexpectedly warm day in February 2008, you see Karl Malden enter an office building. Your tongue-in-cheek campaign to get your home town to host the 2018 Olympics leads to real danger.

**SCORPIO** *(October 24–November 21):* A life of undefined desires. In May 2009, you are rightfully declared innocent following a protracted and highly publicized skyjacking trial. In redecorating your kitchen (year uncertain) you find something that someone who claims to be James Bond wants very much. Ignore the daily horoscope you read in 2025 that says you will be grazed by a speeding fire truck. Keep an eye out for tow trucks, however.

**SAGITTARIUS** *(November 22–December 21):* A career of seemingly linked but ultimately disparate ideas. For a week in the autumn of 2013 you find yourself with an entourage. The weird knocking on your living room wall finally stops just after midnight, April 4, 2015. Ice sports become important—and lucky. Begin getting in shape now (particularly practice the broad jump) for a narrow escape you will have to make while vacationing near sand.

**CAPRICORN** *(December 22–January 19):* You never run out of good last-second solutions. In the spring of 2032 you discover something growing in your yard that eventually attracts worldwide attention. Be sure to wear a belt or carry a length of rope during the summer of 2012. An ill-advised romantic liaison undertaken in October 2009 turns into a humiliating and expensive fiasco. Avoid moustached benefactors.

**AQUARIUS** *(January 20–February 18):* A lifetime of unsatisfactory afternoon naps. A computer error in April 2011 awards you a four-year football scholarship to the University of Oklahoma; you accept at first but later turn it down with a humorous note of explanation. Your mate's purchase of electric hedge clippers leads to unforeseen difficulties. Don't eat anything you find on the sidewalk in 2014–15.

**PISCES** *(February 19–March 20):* The imagined slights continue to cause problems. In November 2008, a bowling partner teaches you how to whistle with your fingers in your mouth. A small metal box you find while snorkeling in 2013 changes your life and makes you a household name in the Sunbelt. As part of the general mid-century madness, in 2049 you lead fellow Pisceans in a march on the astrologers' annual convention to protest your demeaning position at the bottom of the daily horoscope.

## The Right Palm

The right palm is dominated by the life line **A.** The longer this line is, the longer your life will be and the more close and dear friends **G** you will bury. Two other features of the life line are **E,** which indicates that you have a twin brother or sister whom you have never seen (or possibly its half-formed fetus is living inside your own body), and **F,** which represents a series of nagging head colds that besets you during your forties.

Line **B** is the head line. If this line is deeply creased and if it runs from the upper right of the palm to the lower left (as illustrated), it means you have a big head and you think you're all it. If the line runs straight across the palm, it means that if you live long enough (check your life line), you eventually will become a harmless eccentric. A faint line here indicates that you are an airhead. The short lines **I** crossing the head line represent major changes in hairstyles.

Line **C** is the heart line. If it runs straight and true, then so does your love. If there is the slightest curve in it, however, it means that you tend to stray or even that you are undeserving of unswerving devotion. The hash marks **J** along this line represent lewd thoughts you have entertained regarding members of the opposite sex. A branch at the end of the line **H** means either that you will be divorced or that your dog will die before you do.

Line **D** is the fate line. It means that your fate is in your hand. A strong line here indicates that you are a fatalist and you believe that when your number's up, your number's up. Some people have no fate line. This means they have no fate and are free to goof off for the rest of their lives.

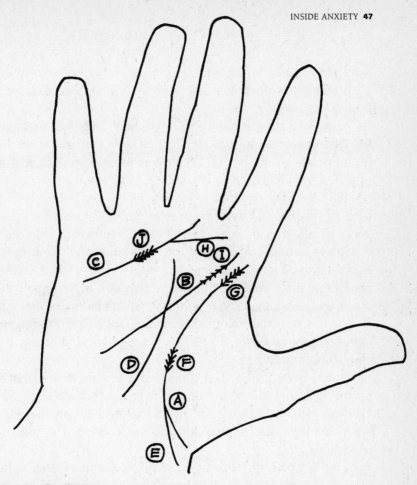

## The Left Palm

The left palm is unjustly ignored by many palm readers, particularly those who ply their trade in saloons. In many ways this palm is much more revealing of one's personality than is the right one.

The first thing to do is to see what letter of the alphabet is formed by the major lines in the palm. This letter will tell you how you like your pizza. If the letter you see is an *M* (as illustrated), it means you like mushrooms and meatballs as a pizza topping; an *A* stands for anchovies, an *S* stands for sausage, and an *N* stands for "nothing" (or just cheese).

Line **A** on the left hand represents how long your *useful* life will last. It corresponds to the life line on your right hand, but it almost always is shorter, because at some point you will no longer be of any use to your family or your society.

Line **B** is your material possession line. If it is long and deep, then so will be your association with and affection for material goods. A fading in the line represents a temporary spell of lethargic consumer activity; a break in the line indicates bankruptcy. Hash marks **G** on the **B** line represent major cash outlays—marks that meet the **B** line but do not cross it indicate palpable purchases (a house, a car, a painting), while marks that cross the **B** line indicate great amounts of money spent for no apparent reason (children's tuition, $500-a-plate political dinners, dog obedience courses).

The meaning of line **C** is contained in a letter that was given to the Pope in 1937 by a group of Belgian schoolchildren who claimed to have been visited by the Blessed Virgin. No Pope since that time has felt that the world is ready for the contents of the letter.

Line **D** represents your willingness to pick up the check after dinner. If it is red and throbbing, it means you should at least *try* to pick up the check every once in a while.

Line **E** represents your political leaning. It should be read from top to bottom. Generally, this line moves from left to right, with a markedly vicious swerve to the right in old age. Abrupt jumps in the direction of the line represent galvanizing issues. Breaks in the line indicate brief flings with third-party politics.

Line **F** is your credit line. Consult it before you consult the **D** line.

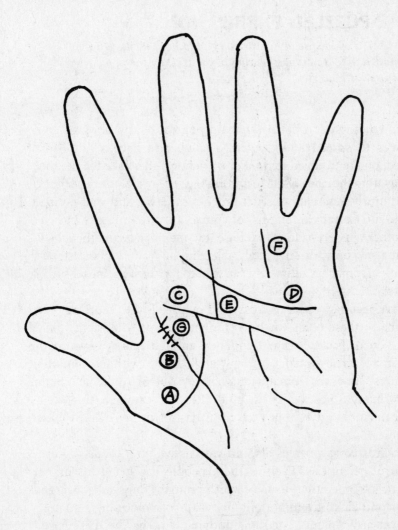

# THE PUZZLED EXPRESSION

*By 1927 a wide-spread neurosis began to be evident, faintly signalled, like a nervous beating of the feet, by the popularity of crossword puzzles.*

—F. SCOTT FITZGERALD

And so crossword puzzles remain popular as the neurosis continues to spread and deepen. The puzzles have a salubrious effect on the troubled mind. For a brief time they take the neurotic away from the cares of the real world (i.e., the rest of the newspaper) and into a sanctuary of strict order, clear laws, and well-defined borders. Certain among us, of course, turn the puzzles into yet another anxiety-ridden exercise by racing against the clock, using ink only, or sneeringly rejecting any offers of assistance. These approaches ultimately can lead to the most profound sort of misery.

A peculiar aspect of crossword puzzles is the recurring clue. Some of these clues, such as "Oriental nurse," "Moslem ruler," or "son of Isaac," occur frequently enough that we eventually learn to write "amah," "emir," and "Esau" without blinking. Others, however, remain tantalizingly out of reach no matter how many times we see the clue. "P.I. tree" can be a tough one, as can "indigo dye," but each of us has his or her own problem clues.

Crossword puzzles also provide us with a curious aggregation of celebrities. Each of these people has made his or her mark in some other, usually worthy pursuit only to be awarded a second claim to immortality by virtue of possessing a strange, vowel-heavy name. The same undying fame has been conferred upon a handful of cities, animals, and natural watercourses as well. So often does the puzzle fancier write down these names that it is easy to forget they are real people and real places. What follows may be considered the charter membership of the Crossword Puzzle Hall of Fame. They *do* have faces, after all. Let us quietly salute each one of them.

1. Prince Ito
2. Arthur Ashe
3. Leon Uris
4. James Agee
5. Sandra Dee
6. Niels H. D. Bohr (*Nobel physicist*)
7. Elia (*Charles Lamb*)
8. Ina Clair
9. Erle Stanley Gardner
10. Eero Saarinen

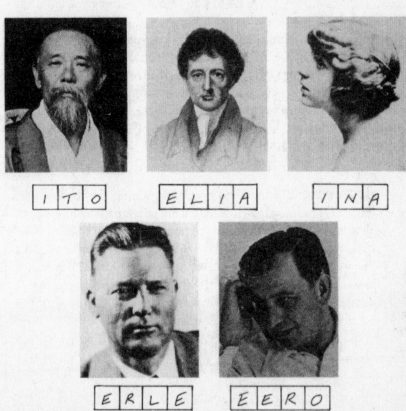

# BIG MONEY IN YOUR SPARE TIME

The act of hoarding being a key neurotic trait, the recent surge in the collectibles market is something that many neurotics have been preparing for all their lives, whether they realized it or not. For years they have been cluttering up closets and basements and garages with old bottles, baseball cards, commemorative plates, comic books, postcards, Coca-Cola trays, and anything else they could get their hands on. Now, in an age when anything that shows the slightest hint of wit or craftsmanship is worth big money, these collectors are sitting pretty.

There is another type of collector, equally neurotic, who is still waiting patiently for his day in the sun. This collector has a somewhat less discerning eye for value, a somewhat less sophisticated notion of what collecting is all about, yet his ardor is real. Since it is difficult for this secondary collector to gather information about his holdings, the following guide should be of some use.

1.  **SUGAR PACKETS.** Not too much happening in this field yet, but the gradual turn toward sugar substitutes makes for a very rosy prospect indeed. Anyone who has a full set of state bird or state flower packets is sitting on at least $1.50, and the value can only go up. The cognoscenti are still hunting down stray packets from the infamous Bicentennial Presidential Series of 1976 in which Dwight Eisenhower was mistakenly given enormous side-whiskers.

2.  **PAPER PLACE MATS.** Instructional mats—"Sam Snead on the Bunker Shot," "Sammy Davis, Jr., on Showmanship," and "Rod McKuen on Sonnets"—remain popular among collectors. Rarer, however, are the "Map of France" mats that were ordered by the New York City restaurant Lutèce only to be

discarded after several weeks' use. Lovers of errata are always on the lookout for the Howard Johnson's kiddie mat gaffe of 1967 in which there was no way out of the maze.

3. **DRINK STIRRERS.** Not the cheap ones that you twist into nasty little knots or chew until the fibers get stuck in your teeth during tense nights out on the town, but the big, breakable plastic ones that have "This is a swanky joint" written all over them and for some reason a little ball down at the business end. All forms of this potentially valuable collectible are becoming rare, but especially ones with penguins or gaudy arrangements of plastic fruit on the top. If you have one that actually has "This is a swanky joint" written all over it, hang on to it.

4. **PENNIES.** Still not too much movement here, but by all means keep hoarding them. Something big is bound to break soon, perhaps even a switchover to a yenlike currency by the United States some time in 2024. Such a switch would make the penny obsolete as legal tender, and naturally very valuable to the serious (over forty thousand pennies saved) collector.

# GETTING THROUGH THE YEAR

The Four Seasons of the Neurotic

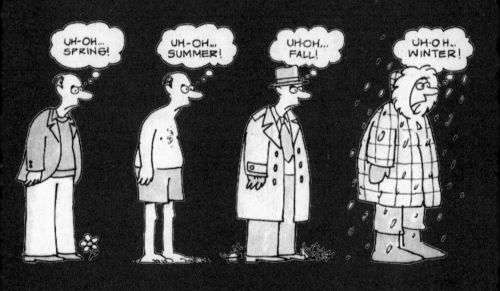

# SUMMER

Summer is a season of sultry menace. All of nature is alive and snapping. Danger lurks in trees and bushes, flits about in the air, patrols the waters, and crawls upon the very earth itself. The chain of life is in a state of bloody fullness, each link protecting its territory, wildly reproducing, blindly gorging itself on the unlucky members of neighboring links.

Neurotics make themselves needlessly susceptible to this festering Grand Guignol by blithely venturing out of doors. Despite bitter past experience, we nose into unfamiliar places in an attempt to commune with nature. We wear fewer clothes. We are, in effect, asking for trouble, and summer is more than prepared to dish it out.

Luckily, while the irritations and worries of summer are staggeringly numerous, most of them are minor; while winter threatens us with isolation, starvation, and death, summer fosters rashes and a lack of pockets. Many of summer's problems are also quite easily avoided. The simple act of staying indoors, for instance, eliminates much that is harmful. If you must go outside, avoid extremely hot places and also shady, cool, moist places and you'll find that things go much more smoothly. Do not exert yourself. Seek comfort at any cost. And, for heaven's sake, don't eat that chicken salad sandwich that's been sitting there in the sun since 11 o'clock this morning.

## Some Facts of Summer

1.  If you punch a shark in the nose, it will get scared and go away.

2.  Never take a shower or use a telephone during a thunder and lightning storm; the lightning will come right down the nozzle or through the receiver and throw you across the room.

3.  Bats are attracted to and get tangled in long hair. Rabies shots are worse than rabies.

4.  Don't touch a beached jellyfish, because it can and will sting you. Use a stick.

5.  The books you find left behind in a rented cottage always include a paperback copy of *The Rise and Fall of the Third Reich*. The pages of these books are yellowed and rippled and tend to fall out in chunks.

6.  Summer colds are worse than winter colds.

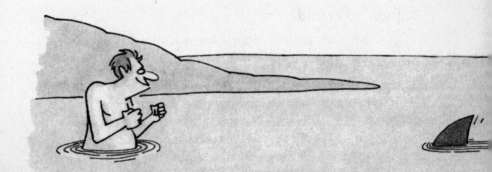

7. If you hold a buttercup up to someone's throat and there is a yellow reflection, it means he or she likes butter. There always is a yellow reflection.

8. Crickets chirp the temperature. You count the number of chirps in a minute and add fourteen, or something like that. European crickets chirp in centigrade.

9. All cottages have enough hot water for only one shower. There never are any dry towels around anyway.

10. No one has ever seen a baby seagull.

## Things Not to Say

1. "I can tread water indefinitely."
2. "These mushrooms are perfectly safe."
3. "I don't burn, I tan."
4. "Let's swim all the way across."
5. "If you don't bother it, it won't bother you."
6. "Poison ivy? I'm immune to it."
7. "Let's see what's under this rotting log."
8. "The diving board wouldn't be here if the water wasn't deep enough."

## Things to Avoid

1. Touching the bottom of the lake with your feet.
2. Feeling sorry for moths after you have killed them.
3. Food at drive-in movies, particularly hamburgers that have been piled under one of those orange lightbulbs.
4. Looking under docks.

5. Getting serious about miniature golf or ski-ball.

6. Cleaning the windshield or radiator grill after a long drive in the country.

7. Testing the power of your lawn mower by running it over large sticks and roots.

8. Holding the firecracker while someone else lights it.

## Disquieting Questions

1. What makes lakeside cottages smell like that?

2. Are they *really* calling for help or are they just fooling around?

3. How does the sand get into the cap of the peanut butter jar?

4. What causes the slime on pool dressing room floors?

5. What mouth disease will you contract if you drink out of that hose?

6. What are the qualifications—if any—of people who check rollercoasters for safety?

7. What goes on inside those thick white webs that grow in the crooks of tree branches (usually in swamps)?

8. Is it really possible to grow a watermelon in your stomach if you accidentally swallow a watermelon seed?

## How to Stuff a Wild Espadrille

You have taken the last swim of the day and now it is time to go home. The beach sand is very hot. You do not want to walk across it barefoot, but you also do not want to put your sandy, gritty feet into your shoes. You are now faced with one of the gnawing dilemmas of summer. You must somehow get two clean feet into two dry shoes while standing in wet sand and water. Here is what you must do:

1.  Carry your shoes to the water's edge. Find a spot where the water is hissing up with enough force to wash your feet but not with enough strength to knock you down. Concentrate your mind. Ignore the fact that people behind you on the beach are watching.

2.  Stand on one foot. Dip the other foot into the ocean and swish it around lightly. If you are unable to stand on one foot, find a jetty that is not covered with slippery green stuff and work from there.

3.  Extract the now clean foot from the water and wave it as violently as you dare in the breeze. Then, with a swift movement, bend forward at the waist and place the correct shoe on this foot. Be careful that you do not absentmindedly drop the other shoe during this deft maneuver.

4.  Hop backward rapidly in the manner of a sandpiper to avoid a suddenly surging wave.

5.  Take a moment to assess the situation. Your shod foot is still in the air. Your anchoring leg is tiring quickly and beginning to wobble. Redouble your concentration.

6.  Lie down.

7.  Prop yourself up on your elbows as if you were casually viewing a sunset, but remember to hold the empty shoe away from the sand.

8.  Using your elbows and your bare foot, crabwalk slowly down toward the water line. Be especially careful here not to get sand in the elastic band of your bathing suit.

9.  When you get to the water, select a wave that will come in

just about right. Dip and extract (numbers 2 and 3 above) and then draw the newly clean foot in toward your chest and place the shoe on it.

10. Continue into a backward somersault (don't get sand in your hair!), stand, turn, and, acknowledging the cheers of the crowd, stroll triumphantly home.

## Cramps Checklist

Of the many fears hammered into us during childhood, one of the most persistent and horrifying is the theory that states that if you go into the water shortly after eating, you will develop stomach cramps and drown. There did not seem to be any way of getting around the fatal nature of this theory: if you went swimming too soon, you died.

The natural neurotic extension of this theory is the question of *how long* one should wait before taking to the water. How can you tell when you're ready? Does how long you have to wait have anything to do with what type of food you have just eaten?

Here is a handy list to post next to the tide tables or the No Running Near the Pool sign. It tells you how long you must wait after eating certain benchmark foods. The times are not approximate, they are exact.

| | |
|---|---|
| Popsicle (any flavor) | 30 seconds |
| Jell-O | 1 minute |
| Jell-O with bananas in suspension | 20 minutes |
| Watercress sandwich | 3½ minutes |
| Martini | 5 minutes |
| Martini with olive | 8 minutes |
| Frozen Milky Way | 12 minutes |
| Burger, fries, Coke | 25 minutes |
| Tuna casserole | 40 minutes |

| Baked beans | 2½ hours |
| Pop-Tarts | 3 hours (each) |
| McDonald's apple pie | Wait till next summer |

## AUTUMN/FALL

This is the only season with two names, and neurotics love both of them more for the associations they bring to mind than for anything that actually happens. They love autumn/fall because it is a time for looking back into the idealized past, a time for wistfulness and profound feelings of loss and bittersweet memories regarding gum erasers, roaring football crowds, and desperate embraces under swirling skies. They love it also because it is a time for jittery glances ahead to the desolation of winter, for gathering and hunkering down (two favored neurotic activities), and for heightened worrying about snow tires, storm windows, insulation, antifreeze, and the like.

There is great comfort to be taken from the death of nature. As the weather worsens there are fewer and fewer reasons to be out and about, fewer diversions that involve hastily drawn directions on tiny scraps of paper. In autumn/fall the focus of concern comes back sharply to where it belongs: yourself. Once again it is perfectly okay to curl up under a blanket on the couch to daydream and drift off. Once again there is ample time for you to reflect upon the fact that you are but a speck in an endless universe. And a cold, rainy day in November is the perfect time for you to lie in bed with a pillow over your head and go over and over how you cowered before a maître d's icy stare while on vacation nine years ago—and to reconstruct the scene so that you come out on top.

Neurotic behavior is not only acceptable in autumn/fall, it is expected.

## Some Facts of Autumn/Fall

1. The more of a hurry you are in, the more school buses you get stuck behind.

2. The people sitting around you at the football game are always better prepared to deal with hunger, thirst, and the weather.

3. Your neighbors' leaves always end up in your yard. Your leaves drop straight down.

4. Indian corn (the kind that people nail to their front doors) is poisonous.

5. Children should not sniff the mimeograph ink on their school test papers. Doing so will lead to a steady deterioration of the brain.

6. The strength of a hurricane is inversely proportional to its advance billing.

7. Many hunters have no idea of what they are doing.

8. Third-party political candidates who are gawky and loud and have bad teeth complain that they are being ignored by the media.

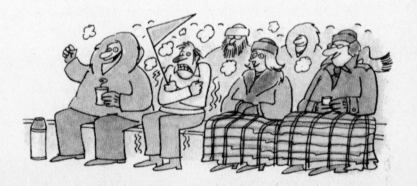

9. Everyone misses the smell of burning leaves. No one does anything about it.

10. It is *not* impossible to ruin a turkey.

## But Hard! What Gale through Yonder Window Blows?

You thought it would be a nice idea to get some fresh air while you slept, so you left the window open last night. At approximately 2:35 A.M., an arctic cold front swept down from Canada and noisily set up shop in your bedroom. At 3:11 A.M., an icy blast knocked a cherished framed photograph off the dresser; you woke up, observed the curtains blowing straight into the room, pulled the blankets tightly over your head, and, knowing you would pay later, went back to sleep. It is now later. Your alarm clock is ringing. The temperature in your room is 19 degrees. Your rigid form clings to a patch of warmth that through some thermodynamic fluke is narrower than you are. You urgently have to go to the bathroom. Movement, even the thought of movement, is agony. It is time to greet the day.

1. With lizard quickness, dart your hand out from under the pillow and turn off the alarm. Your finger will stick to the metal shut-off device. Rip your finger away and bring it back under your chest. Whimper like a little baby.

2. Bring the blanket down to the bridge of your nose and peek out into the room. What you once thought was a comfortable lair has become hostile, alien territory. Wonder why the fool of an architect put the bathroom way over there. Consider it likely that the fool of an architect now lives in Florida. Put your head back under the covers.

3. Spend time considering inventions that could save you from

such discomfort—and make you a millionaire. Perhaps a remote control switch that would turn on the hot water in the shower and fill the house with steam. Think about what you could do with the money. Would you give some away to charity? If so, what charity? What kind of car would you buy? What color? Debate these points. Doze.

4. Alarm goes off again. Climb back to consciousness from a sun-splotched reverie and repeat Step 1, using a different finger. Curse yourself for buying such an alarm clock. Consider that your boss probably is not cowering in bed right now, is probably on the way to work, humming happily. That's why you're not the boss. Curse society.

5. Time to stop the foolish stalling. You've known all along that a warm robe is draped over the back of a chair but that it is just out of reach. Luckily, however, as you stare at the floor thinking of nothing in particular, you notice that the wind has blown down a set of curtains and a curtain rod that *is* in reach. Make dim, apelike calculations. Then use the curtain rod as an extension of the human arm to secure the robe and hoist it to the bed. Rest.

6. Sit up under the blankets, making a crude tent. With a brisk set of thrashing motions, put on the robe. Do not sacrifice proper procedure for speed, however. Undue haste may result in a tangled mess in which you drag all the bedding into the bathroom with you.

7. From the depths of your woolen igloo, think of a particularly high note from any song you know. (The note on the word *glare* in "The Star-Spangled Banner" would be good for this.) Slowly rise from your crouching position, singing the high note. The higher you rise, the louder you sing. At length, you are standing on your bed, screaming.

8. Fling off the blankets, jump off the bed, and "GLLL-AAAAARRRE!!" your way into the bathroom, running at top running-in-the-house speed. Turn on the hot water, strip while running in place, jump in, stop singing.

9. It is while you are at last luxuriating in the steamy clouds that you will remember that all your clothes are back in the bedroom and the window is still open. Immediately put this thought out of mind. Lather up. Close your eyes. Think of a broad expanse of beach, a tropical drink, big brown eyes. Doze.

## How to Make a Jack-o'-Lantern

Generally speaking, neurotics are less likely to begin fretting over this and that as long as they can keep their hands busy. In addition, the sense of "harvest" is very important to the nostalgic side of their characters. Here, we are able to combine both busy-work and a sense of harvest.

After you've selected the pumpkin, brought it home, spread newspapers (perhaps reading over three or four stories you missed when they first appeared two months ago), and chosen your cutting instrument, you will be ready to begin this delightful seasonal task. You will find the pumpkin to be an orange fruit of considerable bulk. Your job is to breathe life into it. In a sense you are an artist, much like Michelangelo contemplating a virgin hunk of marble. Like that lofty predecessor, you are striving for an artistic ideal.

*Michelangelo's ideal*                    *Your ideal*

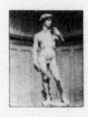                    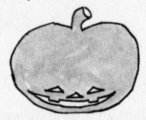

Take your cutting instrument (a knife would be good) and make a "cap" by cutting around the stalk. Remove the cap. Now roll up your sleeves, reach in, and pull out all that disgustingly stringy gunk. Throw away the gunk. Forget about the seeds, too; if you like them, you can find them at a reasonable price in packages in stores.

Now you are ready to go. The eyes should be done first. Don't make them too high or too low or you'll ruin everything.

*Eyes too high*          *Eyes too low*

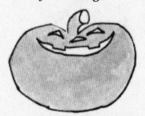          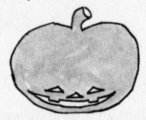

There are three basic types of eyes.

*Regular*                    *Scary*                    *Scared*

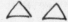                    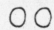

But only one type of nose.

The mouth is a bit trickier, there being the question of teeth. The watchword here is don't get fancy. It's not that important. Again, it's best to stick with one of three choices.

*Harmless smile*　　　　*Toothy grin*　　　　*Scary fangs*

Further tips:

1. No eyeballs.
2. Don't draw on the pumpkin.
3. Don't try eyebrows.
4. No accessories. Hats, pipes, scarves, etc., are for snowmen.
5. Light the candle *after* you put it in the pumpkin.

# WINTER

Neurotics believe that it serves them right to suffer. Some go as far as to believe that they were put on this earth to suffer. Winter is nothing more or less than the perfect excuse for suffering.

Except in those warm regions of the country that have problems of their own, such as characterless residential "loops" and no really good pizza, winter is cold, dark, and windy. The streets are a glaze of ice. Department stores are overheated. The car won't start, and then you make things worse by flooding the engine, and *then* you can't tell when it's not flooded anymore and you can't get back to concentrating on the original problem again.

It is much better just to stay in the house during winter, and that is what many neurotics do (as they do in every other season). It is a time for reading and for brooding over what you have read. It is a time for watching crackerjack old movies on television and wishing they still made them like that. It is a time for reading the newspaper from front page to back and doing the crossword puzzle and even doing the stupid little word jumble puzzles that a three-year-old could do. It is a time for eating out of cans, and listening to radio talk shows, and looking through old letters and yearbooks and photo albums. And all the time, deep down inside, you are suffering. It is a wonderful time.

## Some Facts of Winter

1. Stale odors collect in the house. You can't smell them, but others can.

2. The man who runs the little sidewalk stand where you buy hotdogs spends his winters in Acapulco.

3. The Super Bowl never lives up to the pregame hoopla.

4. There is no such thing as American flu.

5. If you begin feeding the birds, don't stop or they will all die and blame you.

6. Hypothermia strikes without warning and often is fatal. You can get it by just going out to check the mailbox.

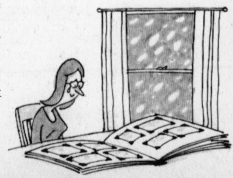

7. If you fall through the ice, you have about three seconds to get out alive.

8. There are more snow tire commercials on television than are necessary.

9. People secretly enjoy getting holiday cards with Xeroxed newsletters in them, even though they say they don't.

10. You never have windshield solvent when you really need it.

## Things Not to Say

1. "Don't worry, I have a natural sense of direction."

2. "It's Grandpa's turn to shovel the snow."

3. "It's cold, but it's a *dry* cold."

4. "Christmas always makes me sad."

5. "You stay here. I'll go out and look for help."

6. "I'll stay here. You go out and look for help."

## Things to Avoid

1. French-kissing under the mistletoe while everyone is watching.

2. Going ski jumping for the first time.

3. People who wear "Kiss me, I'm Irish" buttons on St. Patrick's Day.

4. Expecting mail on Valentine's Day.

5. Saying, "Downhill skiing is too commercialized" when actually you're just scared.

6. Having a frank conversation with the boss during the office Christmas party.

7. Fake tanning agents that turn your skin a ghastly orange.

8. Wearing your pajamas under your regular clothes.

## New Year's Eve

No one much likes New Year's Eve. More specifically, no one much likes New Year's Eve parties, either giving them or going to them. Yet every year there it is (December 31), there it is (the party), and there you go (to it). You think that if you get drunk enough, you may be able to enjoy yourself, but usually the dread is too much to overcome. The dread, that is, of funny hats and noisemakers, of everyone gathered around the television (someone *always* turns it on) at five minutes to midnight, of sour saxophones playing "Auld Lang Syne," of another year down the drain. If there is a worse way of starting a new year than with cheap champagne, forced gaiety, a throbbing hangover, and an endless procession of college football games, it is hard to imagine what it would be. And yet the pressure is so great to partake in all of it that we usually give in without a third or fourth thought.

The alternatives, of course, are even more chilling. To spend the night by yourself is unthinkable and perhaps even suicidal. To spend it among strangers at a lounge or a nightclub with a manic emcee at the helm is desperate and expensive. The only way of getting around the problem is to be madly in love, a prospect that is chancy to say the least.

The trouble with neurotics giving the party is that they take New Year's Eve too seriously. They cannot imagine that it is just another night and just another party, no matter how often they tell themselves that this is so. It's got to be a memorable time and everything has to go perfectly or all is lost. If anyone is having a bad time or is visibly bored, the neurotic host is personally responsible and the party (maybe even the whole coming year) is a washout. If anyone leaves early, it is a slap in the face and may (probably will) trigger a landslide of early departures. Is the music not right? Change it constantly. The food not being eaten?

Bring out more and more and more. No one dancing? Begin badgering close friends.

At the stroke of midnight, when everyone is shouting and kissing and guzzling bubbly, the neurotic host or hostess can be found off to the side of the room, accepting a few perfunctory pecks, but with eyes fixed on the guests, certain of the hollowness of the laughter and cheers, promising never to go to or hold a New Year's Eve party again. And thinking that it would be better to clean everything up before going to bed than it would be to face this mess in the morning.

## Christmas Countdown

**DECEMBER 27.** Buy Christmas cards and ornaments and wrapping paper for next year at half price.

**FEBRUARY 7.** Buy your first Christmas present while visiting Myrtle Beach, South Carolina.

**MAY 16.** Buy your second Christmas present from a door-to-door salesman you feel sorry for.

**NOVEMBER 20.** Start dropping hints about what type of presents you could really use.

**NOVEMBER 28.** Buy more cards and ornaments and wrapping paper because you can't remember where you put the ones you bought last year.

**DECEMBER 3.** Spend a day in bed going through all the catalogues, wishing you had the money to buy the nicer things, hoping that someone will splurge on you.

**DECEMBER 12.** Start out on the round of holiday parties.

**DECEMBER 14.** Vow to go on a diet right after Christmas (or maybe the New Year).

**DECEMBER 15.** Complain about the overcommercialization of Christmas.

**DECEMBER 16.** State emphatically what you want for presents.

**DECEMBER 17.** Start hoping against hope for a white Christmas.

**DECEMBER 18.** Buy a Christmas tree that costs what your grandfather got for a weekly salary when he first started working.

**DECEMBER 19.** Receive a Christmas card with a personal note signed "Dan and Nancy." You can't think of anyone named Dan *or* Nancy, much less Dan *and* Nancy.

**DECEMBER 20 (8 P.M.).** Begin stringing popcorn for the tree.

**DECEMBER 20 (8:35 P.M.).** Give up stringing popcorn.

**DECEMBER 21.** Witness a salesclerk at a crowded department store suffer a nervous breakdown and smash a vase over a customer's head.

**DECEMBER 22.** Send cards to the people you forgot about.

**DECEMBER 23.** Realize you haven't bought any presents since May 16. Race around from store to store with nothing in mind. Buy nothing.

**DECEMBER 24.** Buy all your presents at a large drugstore at 9 P.M.

**DECEMBER 25.** Smile bravely and try to say, "Thank you" as if you really meant it.

## SPRING

It is hard for even the confirmed neurotic to ignore the glory of spring, but it can be done. Indeed, dark thoughts and anxiety can make a fascinating counterpoint to a world that is all aborning and atwit.

The main thing to remember about spring is that summer is close at hand, then fall, and then it will be winter again almost before you realize it. Add to this the common belief that each year whizzes by more quickly than the last (by the time you are eighty you barely have enough time to unwrap your birthday presents—if you get any—before you turn eighty-one) and you will find yourself in a dither that even the most insistent robin or daffodil will be unable to untangle.

The spring is the time for other people to fall in love, to hatch grand, ambitious plans, to get themselves back in shape. Neurotics, meanwhile, continue along much as before. They dream of a love that is unattainable, they produce grand plans but they do not hatch them, and they either put off getting into shape until tomorrow or, if they do start running, they can't stop.

Spring is difficult. It is a hurdle that must be cleared. Just don't let it get to you.

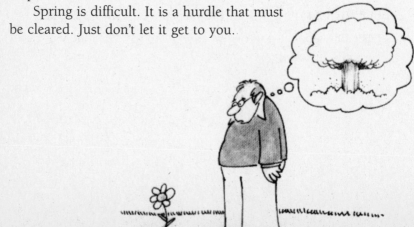

## Some Facts of Spring

1. Crocuses come out too early every year, as do all the hopes associated with them.

2. An honorary degree and thirty cents will buy you a cup of coffee.

3. Kids who go to Fort Lauderdale always manage to find beds of their own to sleep in.

4. Tornadoes strike mobile home parks far more often than mere chance would permit.

5. Wedding photographers are becoming more obtrusive with each passing year.

6. It's people such as you who are most abused by the income tax system.

7. Baby ducks and chickens are treated with fiendish cruelty by the children who get them for Easter.

8. Baseball players don't know how lucky they are.

9. You can be thrown into jail for killing (even accidentally) a praying mantis.

10. New Year's resolutions are made to be broken.

## The Neurotic's Beaufort Scale

Early spring is a season of wind, and wind is troubling to the easily distracted mind. First of all, what is wind? Where does it come from, and where does it go? Is the breeze that today blows our hair the wrong way across our heads (just as the photographer clicks the shutter) the very same breeze that hundreds of years ago riffled through the beard of Balboa as he stood surveying the Pacific?

These are numbing questions, and they can be answered only in ways that are not understood. More to the point is the fact that wind is simply a nagging feature of nature, almost never welcome, always beyond our control. Words such as *fickle* and *capricious* are used to describe it, and these words rebel against everything the neurotic holds dear to heart.

Luckily for us, however, even the wind has been broken down and categorized by man. The Beaufort scale was devised in 1805 by British naval officer Sir Francis Beaufort. With some emendation the scale can be of use.

| *Beaufort number* | *Miles per hour* | *Neurotic's description* |
| --- | --- | --- |
| 0 | Up to 1 | The calm before the storm |
| 1 | 1 to 3 | What happens when you take the sailboat out |
| 2 | 4 to 7 | Leaves begin to clatter annoyingly |
| 3 | 8 to 12 | Bring the card game inside |
| 4 | 13 to 18 | Danger for secretly balding men |
| 5 | 19 to 24 | The picnic turns into a fiasco |
| 6 | 25 to 31 | What happens when you take the canoe out |
| 7 | 32 to 38 | Doleful moaning in the eaves |
| 8 | 39 to 46 | Cancel all plans |
| 9 | 47 to 54 | Growing sense of panic |
| 10 | 55 to 63 | Finally get to use the candles |
| 11 | 64 to 72 | Have to go to the store for matches |
| 12 | 73 to 136 | Why don't they ever name a hurricane after me? |

## Spring Cleaning

There are neurotics who are obsessed with tidiness and cleanliness (and for whom Felix Unger of *The Odd Couple* stands as a shining, sparkling, spotless beacon). These people need not worry about the ritual of spring cleaning, because dirt long ago gave up the fight and moved out permanently to some more accommodating household. With the coming of spring these remarkable characters can be seen engaged in more arcane chores, such as polishing the tailpipe of the family car, replacing the soil and grass in the backyard with Astroturf, or scrubbing skidmarks off the street. We all know such people. We probably have one in the family.

For the rest of us, however, spring cleaning is a basic, strenuous pain. We are presumed to have been lying around in a vaguely self-satisfied stupor all winter, spilling things and not wiping them up, exuding bad odors, perhaps even bedding down on piles of hay with goats and poultry. Then, at some point in early spring, we are overcome by an urge to begin cleaning. This urge usually coincides with something else we are supposed to do that is much more important, such as finding a job or filing income tax returns.

In any case, the task need not be quite as hard as it seems. The first step is to pick a sunny weekday, with birds chirping, brooks babbling, and so forth. Then, following a nourishing breakfast, try the following:

1. With childish glee, rush from room to room and open all the windows. After opening the last one that hasn't been soldered shut by the mysterious forces of nature, stand before it and breathe dramatically.

2. Put on a sweater.

3. Go look under the sink to make sure that all your cleaning

agents are in order. Admire the colorful array of fine, nearly full bottles and jugs. Read several of the frightening warnings on the labels.

4. Check your clothes closet. In a corner you will see a pair of shoes you bought years ago but never had the guts to wear in public. Put them on. Walk around the room. Put them back.

5. Time for dusting. Run the cuff of a shirt you are not wearing across the dust cover of your stereo turntable. See how the plastic almost shimmers. Test the effectiveness of this newly dusted component by putting on a record.

6. Do a totally uninhibited dance until the record is over.

7. While looking in the refrigerator for something to eat, you will find toward the rear of the bottom shelf an unmarked glass jar containing a murky, unidentifiable substance. If you don't throw it in the garbage now, it will be there *next* spring. Throw it away.

8. Near the jar you will find the open box of baking soda. Does it still look potent or does it look used up? Try to figure out how you are supposed to know when your baking soda is used up. Sniff it. Study the box to see if it contains an answer to your dilemma. Read the entire box. Chuckle over the many odd uses of the product. Pour the baking soda down the drain. Wonder why having a freshened drain is so satisfying—almost thrilling.

9. Spend the rest of the day rearranging things. Rearrange your socks alphabetically, according to color. Rearrange your food according to the expiration dates on the packages. Rearrange the things in your closet according to how much they cost. Think of your own madcap ways of rearranging things.

10. With a strong feeling of a job well done, drift from room to room and shut each window. Your house is now clean.

## Dead Skunk Odor Graph

It is in the spring that all the blessed beasts and insects take their first timid baby steps onto a road of life that is also filled with traffic. One of the most vivid signs that this process once again is taking place in the woods is the aroma of a skunk that has been flattened by a speeding auto. The odor (which never really goes away completely) can be depicted this way:

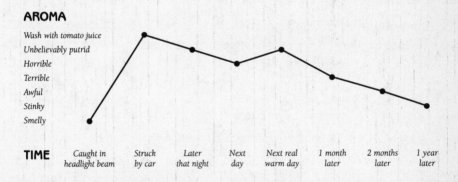

AROMA

Wash with tomato juice
Unbelievably putrid
Horrible
Terrible
Awful
Stinky
Smelly

TIME    Caught in      Struck     Later      Next      Next real    1 month    2 months    1 year
        headlight beam  by car    that night  day      warm day     later      later       later

# "TRESPASSERS WILL BE PROSECUTED"

### The Neurotic at Home

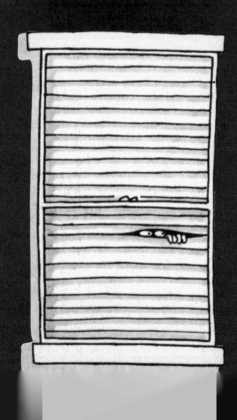

There is no place like home for the neurotic; whether it be a house or an apartment, it is the center of what little control you have over your life. At home you know which electrical outlets work and which are broken, you know the safest place to go to cower during a thunderstorm, you think you know where the pliers are. More important, if you like to put ketchup or even catsup on your scrambled eggs, fine: at home you can put as much on them as you like. You don't have to answer the phone even if someone (you know who) rings it forty-seven times before hanging up. You can lie in bed all day drinking sherry and playing old records that make you cry. You are allowed to cut the cheese whenever you want to. In short, you can be your-self at home, and *no one can do anything about it.*

As pleasant as this may sound, it is not meant to imply that the home is a paradise. Rather, it is a familiar sort of purgatory. It is a place where the runaway problems of life in general are replaced by problems that are specific and predictable. If, for instance, you are in way over your head at work and you lose the Fegley account, it can be oddly comforting to come home and kill a mouse. Or if a pushy salesclerk bullies you into buy-ing something you don't need or want, you can always go home and refuse to return a ball that has been hit into your yard by the neighborhood punk and then threaten to call the police when he sasses you back.

Home is the neurotic's safe harbor. It is there, amid the familiar patterns and the pleasantly sagging springs, that you have best arrayed your defenses against the storm tides of life. It is there that you have put your indelible stamp on everything and everyone. Finally, it is at home that the neurotic can let his or her peculiar personality run wild—and find that people understand. Or at least say that they understand.

# THE TWO MOST IMPORTANT ROOMS

If neurotics were forced to say which room in the house they would want to bring along with them to a desert island, most would choose the kitchen or the bedroom. (A few would pick the bathroom, but it wouldn't take them long to see just how wrong they were.) The kitchen and the bedroom are essential retreats for the neurotic, the former being a key base of mindless activity and the latter being a key base of mindless passivity.

## The Kitchen

Actually, if they thought about it, most neurotics would take the kitchen to the desert island because it would be easier to get all that sand off the floor. That aside, however, the kitchen offers much else. It is warm there, first of all. It is where the food is. It usually is well lighted. And, curiously, there is a mysterious force associated with the kitchen that just seems to draw neurotics into it. If you don't think that this is true, check the kitchen the next time you go to a fairly large party at someone's house. The neurotics will be in there sitting on the counters, chatting, poking their noses into the refrigerator.

## A TYPICAL NEUROTIC'S KITCHEN

1. Clock on the stove doesn't work.

2. Bulletin board. String for pencil but no pencil. Several phone numbers with no names to go with them and a few out-of-date invitations.

3. Magnets on the refrigerator door—ladybugs or other cheerful insects.

4. Stove fan turned on most of the time for the soothing drone.

5. Switch for garbage disposal that everyone turns on thinking it is for a light.

6. Favorite coffee cup.

7. Emergency phone numbers posted by telephone.

8. Poison antidote chart on inside of door under sink.

9. Cooking implements (wok, chafing dish, dry air popcorn popper, electric knife) bought and then used only once.

10. Drawer containing trading stamps.

11. Drawer containing masking tape, rubber bands, scissors, string, twine, thumbtacks, ball and jacks, glue, paste, bus schedule, coupons, dice, picture hangers, playing cards, Band-Aids, screwdriver, extension cords, socket adapters, birthday candles, assorted clasps, brads, screws, hooks, hinges, and nails, jar lids, flashlight, cheap combs, thread, crayons, keys, Magic Markers with points smashed down, coins, matches, potholders, electrical tape, emery board, glitter, toothpicks, a pocket astrology book, an old yellowed roll of adhesive tape that no one had good enough finger-nails to get started again, a broken meat thermometer, booster tickets, and, way in the back, a three-year-old Lions Club raffle ticket and a drink stirrer from a fancy Polynesian restaurant.

12. A kitchen witch.

13. Room freshener disguised as an owl.

14. An industrial-size fire extinguisher.

15. Cabinet full of canned goods in case of natural disaster or nuclear attack.

16. Charcoal filter attached to water faucet.

17. Smoke detector.

18. A cute cover for the toaster.

19. In the refrigerator: a baking soda holder disguised as a penguin.

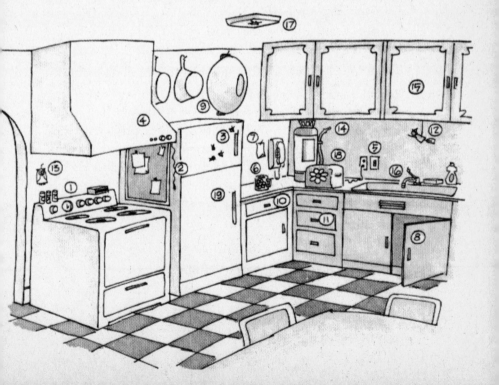

## The Bedroom

The bedroom is where neurotics go when they don't have anything else to do. More specifically, they go to bed. But when neurotics go to bed they are not necessarily going to sleep; they are merely "going to bed for a while." This might mean they are planning to read, listen to the radio, plot out certain strategies, sift through old letters, sneak chocolate chip cookies, fantasize, or just lie there face down in the pillow thinking about nothing at all. Neurotics pass a remarkable amount of time doing just these things, none of which would be nearly so much fun without the privacy of the bedroom to surround them with.

### A TYPICAL NEUROTIC'S BEDROOM

1.  Glow-in-the-dark telephone dial.
2.  Bedside radio (by far the most reliable appliance in the house).
3.  Mysterious light switch that doesn't turn anything on or off.
4.  Bedside table drawer (medicine cabinet annex) containing nose spray, throat lozenges, nail clippers, Kleenex, fast-acting indigestion tablets, rounded scissors, a tawdry paperback thriller, three pieces of toffee, a candle, a shopping receipt once used as a bookmark, a picture postcard, and a small jewelry box containing bobby pins, ticket stubs, two safety pins, a metal chain, and a postage stamp.
5.  Glass of water.
6.  A comforter that cost a fortune but was well worth it.
7.  An electric blanket (under the comforter).
8.  Smoke detector.
9.  A rope ladder.

10. The window that is always accidentally left open during violent rainstorms.

11. A heating pad.

12. Books. One that you have been trying to plow through for eight months (*The Gulag Archipelago, Of Time and the River, Ulysses*) and one that you actually are reading (*The Book of Lists*, the Spiegel catalogue, *Horton Hears a Who*).

13. Lamp with three-way bulb that doesn't work properly.

14. Mirror with reminders taped to it ("Dentist Tuesday," "Gift for Helen!!!").

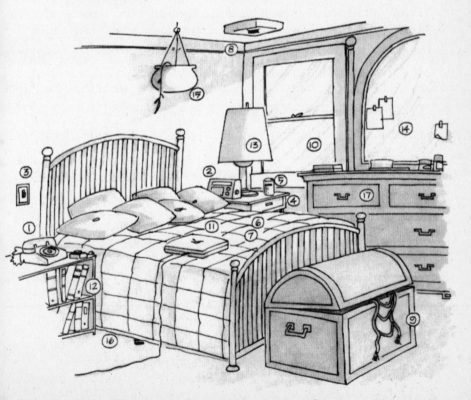

15. Plant that seems to be dying no matter where you put it or what you do with it.

16. Under the bed: two unmatched socks, a pin for an eyeglass hinge, distressing dust build-up, one Oreo.

17. In the underwear drawer: lavender or cedar sachet.

## One Night in the Life of a Neurotic

From time to time, of course, the bedroom is also used for sleeping, or what the neurotic accepts as sleeping. Very rarely does the night pass without incident:

**11:06 P.M.** In bed and ready for sleep. Eyeshades on. Earplugs in to block out the sound of a dripping faucet. Thinking about finances.

**11:16 P.M.** Turning pillow over to "cool" side. Still thinking about finances.

**11:40 P.M.** Switching the radio to an all-night talk show.

**12:05 A.M.** Try putting head at other end of bed. Thinking about idealized vacation spots.

**12:16 A.M.** Align body more properly with gravitational field.

**12:43 A.M.** Asleep at last. Fetal position, with thumb in mouth, lying across the bed.

**1:25 A.M.** Nightmare about not being able to find college classroom where a big exam is being held. Head under pillow.

**1:34 A.M.** Awake in cold sweat, sitting up in bed, as professor turns out to be Bert Parks.

**1:55 A.M.** Resume sleep. Fetal, thumb in mouth.

**3:16 A.M.** Dream about sliding into third base in Yankee Stadium in World Series, smashing into lamp, radio, and glass of water.

**3:56 A.M.** Third baseman for Yanks turns out to be Monica Vitti. Smiling, hugging pillow.

**5:05 A.M.** Wake up with feeling that a stranger is in the house. Lying down, peeking from under eyeshades.

**5:06 A.M.** Resume sleep.

**6:35 A.M.** Alarm ringing, birds chirping, sound of cars outside window, etc. Still asleep.

**7:00 A.M.** Still asleep.

**9:15 A.M.** Still asleep.

# TOOLS FOR COPING: THE WHOLE NEUROTIC'S HOUSEHOLD CATALOGUE

There are other rooms in the house besides the kitchen and the bedroom, and they must be properly outfitted with items that help the neurotic get along in the world. There also are a number of items that are heartily recommended for the neurotic's personal use so that he or she may more easily fend off incipient stress and doubt. Our laboratories endorse the following:

1. **THE WHITE-NOISE BOX.** A product made exclusively for neurotics, this box emits an inoffensive droning noise that is meant to block out potentially maddening sounds such as rustling leaves, dogs barking in the distance, and someone trying to jimmy open the front door. A necessity for those who seek the ambience of the womb in later life.

2. **EYESHADES.** So that not even the tiniest sliver of light can intrude upon the innocent dreams of night. Particularly useful if you dream you are a guest panelist on *What's My Line?*

3. **AN ATOMIZER.** Fill it with anything you may want to spray into your throat. One of the great tools for self-coddling.

4. **GIGANTIC CROSSWORD PUZZLE.** Hang it on the wall in the kitchen or the bathroom and you will always have something to do when you would otherwise go out of your mind with boredom.

5. **TELEPHONE ANSWERING MACHINE.** Neurotics are certain that the telephone rings constantly whenever they happen to leave the house and, moreover, that most of the missed calls are critically important. The purchase and installation of an answering machine will prove both of those theories to be incorrect.

6. **A SUN VISOR FOR THE SUN VISOR.** Driving directly into the setting or rising sun can be a very upsetting experience. This handy tinted attachment hooks onto your car's regular sun visor and, combined with sunglasses and a tinted windshield, makes it seem like it's always dusk.

7. **NOSE PLUGS.** The use and display of these plugs help neurotics spot each other at crowded beaches and pools. Better yet, they have no known medical benefit.

8. **RETURN ADDRESS STICKERS.** There's no really good reason why neurotics comprise the natural market for these items, but they do.

9. **COFFEE CUP WITH YOUR NAME ON IT.** A must for home and office. Neurotics abhor the idea of drinking out of someone else's cup and believe that theirs makes the coffee taste better.

10. **GIANT THERMOMETER.** Neurotic people usually are very anxious about the weather—they talk about it all the time, they keep their ears glued to the radio for weather updates, they get all worked up over approaching big storms. They also

somehow feel secure if they know exactly what the temperature is outside. The larger the thermometer, the more "official" the temperature seems.

11. **JAPANESE BALL MASSAGE.** For the relief of psychosomatic aches and pains. Actually, any massage device from a foreign country is okay.

12. **MONEY BELT.** Worn so that the big-city creeps and crooks won't spot you for a rube when you roll into town. Always keep a little cash in your wallet, though, so the crooks don't shoot you for disappointing them.

13. **VIBRATING FOOT BATH.** Ironically, "tired" feet can keep you awake at night. This nicely humming and rippling item should clear up the problem.

14. **PEDOMETER.** Why should you obsessively count your steps from place to place when you can just carry this little item to do the job for you? Great for neurotic joggers who must know to the nearest foot just how far they've run so they can enter the distance onto the little chart they keep in the bedroom.

15. **RUBBER STAMP ASSORTMENT.** Make a mighty impression on friend and enemy alike with your own distinctive mark. Stamp "Have a nice day" on letters to friends or "Get lost" on letters you send back to collection services. Also, stars, animals, hex signs, and dancing fruit in any color and style.

16. **CAR CUSHION/MASSAGER.** A longtime favorite of neurotics, this device gets air to the otherwise suffocating small of your back as you drive. With the plug-in device, it also can be made to give you a gentle, soothing massage until you are so relaxed that you doze off and careen down a steep embankment.

17. **SCENTED DRAWER LINING.** For a few pennies more, all the drawers in your house can smell like fruit salad or a pine forest.

18. **SOFT TOILET SEAT.** Why did it take so long for someone to invent this? A must.

19. **MAGNETIC EXTRA KEY.** Neurotics have trouble with keys. They either lose them or lock them in the car or don't have the right one at the right time. This nifty device allows you to attach extra keys to the mailbox, auto fender, front porch light, you name it.

20. **SPILL-PROOF DRINK CUP.** Is there anything that gets you more ticked off than spilling hot coffee all over yourself as you hurtle down the expressway at 6:30 in the morning? Now you can be as content as an infant drinking its morning formula out of a baby bottle.

21. **WATER CUSHIONS FOR YOUR FEET.** Simply insert these water-filled pads into your shoes and slosh your troubles away. Amazing "water action" softens corns and calluses, keeps toenails fresh and clean, and keeps between-toes regions free from disgusting foreign matter *while* giving your feet a minimassage at no additional cost.

22. **ELEPHANT BAROMETER.** Place this little fella near a window and he'll turn pink if a storm is coming and blue if the weather is going to clear up, or possibly vice versa.

23. **ROOM HUMIDIFIER.** If you use up more than one stick of lip balm a week, you might consider shelling out plenty for this item. Keeps your lips kissably moist and your hands from getting scaly and red.

# YOUR NEUROTIC HOUSEHOLD QUESTIONS ANSWERED

1. **Q.** What will happen if I use laundry detergent to wash my hands?

   **A.** Probably nothing, but why risk it?

2. **Q.** What happened to those lightbulbs that were supposed to last forever?

   **A.** They're still being tested.

3. **Q.** I always get mixed up between eaves and gables and am afraid of using the wrong word in otherwise informed conversation. What's the difference?

   **A.** There isn't any—they're just French and English words for the same thing. We call them dormers here in the U.S.A.

4. **Q.** How many throw cushions are too many for the average couch?

   **A.** Forty-seven.

5. **Q.** Has an adult ever gotten trapped inside an abandoned refrigerator or suffocated in a dry cleaning bag?

   **A.** No.

6. **Q.** What the hell is grout?

   **A.** Grout is a drink that Dutch sailors used to take along on transoceanic voyages to help ward off scurvy.

7. **Q.** What is the correct way to board up windows to protect against hurricane damage?

   **A.** Use a hammer and nails *before* the hurricane strikes.

8. **Q.** Any final judgment on Teflon yet?

   **A.** Not yet.

9. **Q.** Why are those things on roofs called weather vanes? They don't tell you what the weather's going to be like; they just tell you which way the wind is blowing. Shouldn't they be called wind vanes?

   **A.** Yes, they should.

10. **Q.** We just moved into a house with an intercom system that is broken. It made us realize that we've never seen one that worked properly. Has there ever been one that has worked properly?

    **A.** Yes, but the people who owned it never used it anyway. They called one another by merely raising their voices a bit. It didn't kill them.

# LOCUS NEUROTICUS

Everyone knows about the accidents around the house and around town that regularly claim lives and plenty of column inches in the local paper. What we may be less aware of are the daily occurrences that gradually turn us into neurotics. Such occurrences, taken individually, do not seem like much, but when they happen day in and day out for twenty or thirty years, they really can take their toll.

## Petty Aggravations in the Home That Will Eventually Drive You Crazy

1. **EMPTY ICE TRAYS.** You believe in stockpiling and making sure that there always is enough of everything, but no one else does. From the looks of things, you'd think that refilling

an ice tray required an advanced degree (except that people with advanced degrees are among the worst offenders). You eventually learn that if you don't want to have to skim tiny ice slivers off the top of sluggishly freezing cube slots, you'd better just go out and buy a ten-pound bag.

2. **JUST MISSING THE TELEPHONE.** This happens so often that it is unbelievable. You are outside with an armload of groceries or in the shower or otherwise indisposed when suddenly you realize that the phone is ringing. The critical mistake is that you always freeze for a moment to *make sure* that it's ringing or that it is *your* phone. *Then* you sprint, but it's too late. The one ring that you squandered is the one you needed. Every time.

3. **REFERRING TO LAST WEEK'S TV LISTINGS.** There isn't much happening, so you turn to the television listings to see what's on. You correctly page through to Tuesday and are delighted to find a special on coed nude wrestlers from California high schools. You eagerly switch to the right channel only to find a panel discussion on recreational boating safety. You discover that you have mistakenly referred to the guide for last week, which no one had the wit to throw away. The twinge you feel takes about five minutes off your life.

4. **RUNNING OUT OF TOILET PAPER.** You might not mind using paper towels or cocktail napkins or the pages of *Boys' Life,* but why should your guests have to? If grocery stores piled toilet paper rather than candy and sensational tabloids at the checkouts, this problem never would arise.

5. **GETTING TUNA FISH IN THE MAYONNAISE.** Far worse than getting jelly in the peanut butter. The spot of tuna begins to fester and spread a repulsive brown stain. Lunch is ruined. The whole day is ruined.

6. **MISINTERPRETING A SWEEPSTAKES NOTICE.** "You are a win-ner!!" it says on the envelope, and, despite yourself, for just a few seconds you believe it. You are a sucker.

7. **NO PENS THAT WORK OR PENCILS WITH POINTS (AND NOTHING TO WRITE ON) WHEN YOU HAVE TO TAKE AN IMPORTANT PHONE MESSAGE.** So, after rushing around the house opening and slamming drawers, you come back to the phone (convinced that the caller thinks you're a jerk) and scratch out the message with a key on the desktop or (if you are lucky) write it on the back of your electric bill with a stub of a pencil from a miniature golf course.

8. **NO TOWELS IN THE BATHROOM.** This always is discovered after you have showered or bathed, at about the same point when someone knocks at the front door.

## Petty Aggravations around Town That Will Eventually Drive You Crazy

1. **CHOOSING THE WRONG LINE.** It happens at banks, at grocery stores, and at tollbooths: you pick the slowest-moving line. If you get on what clearly is the shortest line at the grocery store, for instance, the customer in front of you turns out to have purchased at least one item that no one knows the price of. With one eye you watch the endless consultations among supermarket personnel while with the other eye you watch the woman with sixty-three items who would've been ahead of you had you chosen the other line march out the door.

2. **CRAZY PEOPLE ARE DRAWN TO YOU.** No matter how crowded the sidewalk or the train station might be, the crazy person

finds you and comes over to you and starts talking to you about the brain police, or whatever the problem is.

3. **PARALLEL PARKING.** People stop walking or talking and turn to watch as you attempt to parallel park the car. They don't ever do this for anyone else.

4. **TRYING TO FIND OUT THE TIME.** As you are driving toward a bank with an alternating time-temperature sign on it, you decide you would like to know the time. Unfortunately, the sign is now in the temperature mode, which it holds until you draw abreast of the bank. Then it switches to the temperature-in-centigrade mode. By now you have driven past the bank and are risking your life by craning around and sticking your head out the window. When the time is finally shown, you have to try to read it through the rearview mirror so that it is backward and upside down and everything else. You end up having no idea what time it is.

5. **AT THE MOVIES.** The person seated behind you has come to the theater not to watch the film, but rather to rotate the contents of six paper bags.

6. **FORGETTING THE MOST IMPORTANT THING.** Planning a turkey dinner? Buy all the trimmings but forget about the turkey. Going to a play? Forget the tickets. Going abroad? Forget your passport. Things always to forget: the corkscrew, the flashlight, the bottle opener, the directions, the insect repellent, your sweater, an umbrella, the letter you meant to mail.

7. **THE FAMILIAR FACE.** There is someone who goes to the same parties you do, to the same restaurants or bars, whom you see, it seems, just about everywhere you go. You have no idea of who this person is. Occasionally this person will call

you by your first name. When this happens you say, "Hi there!" and pretend that you are in a hurry.

8. **DRIVING BEHIND SOMEONE WHO HAS THE DIRECTIONAL BLINKER BLINKING BUT WHO DOES NOT TURN.** Morons are everywhere, of course, but why do they so often end up driving in front of you? As you finally pull even with these people and try to indicate that they have their blinker on, you invariably are met with a polite smile on a face that is so blank and simple it gives you goose pimples.

# ARE YOU NEUROTIC?

One of the easiest ways to tell if you are a neurotic is to take a look at your house or apartment, your yard, your car, and the way you handle the chores that have to do with them. You qualify as a genuine item if you find yourself in agreement with eight of the following:

## Your House

1. You shovel the walk (or sweep it with a broom) one or more times while the snow is still falling.

2. You believe that good fences make good neighbors.

3. You have an "interesting" or "artistic" mailbox.

4. You are among the very first every year to put up Christmas lights and decorations, and you don't take the wreath off the front door until mid-March.

5. You have a Don't Turn in This Driveway sign out by the street.

6. You have the family initial on the front screen door.

7. You have the largest woodpile for miles around.

8. You use an edger to separate your lawn from the sidewalk.

9. You have covered one or more rocks on your property with whitewash.

10. You figure that the cost of one tomato grown in your garden is at least three times the cost of one tomato bought in a grocery store.

## Your Apartment

1. Your holiday decorations are directed at people outside on the street or in other apartments rather than at people who come to visit you.

2. You watch television all the time but have only a tiny black-and-white set that doesn't pick up any channels clearly (even though you live right in the middle of the city).

3. You hate to have the elevator stop at a strange floor while you are riding in it.

4. Most of the photographs on display are of yourself.

5. You have been living in the apartment for three years or more but don't know any of your neighbors except to say "Hello" to.

6. You have plenty of complaints about the management, but you don't join the tenants' association because you feel the people in it are obnoxious and just looking out for themselves.

7. You live with other people and you buy your own food and put name tags on things such as milk cartons and tubs of cottage cheese.

8. You insist that the view makes up for the fact that there rarely is hot water and the heat always goes out on the coldest nights of the year.

9. You feel that everyone else in the building knows everything about you even though none of them has ever spoken to you personally.

10. You are sick of just "throwing money down the drain" and would like to buy a place of your own. You have felt this way for more than five years.

## Your Car

1. You wash and wax your car to the point where friends and neighbors remark about it.

2. You have a car that is more than twelve years old but in nearly perfect condition.

3. You have a small, scented pine tree made of cardboard hanging from the dashboard.

4. You have a horn that plays the first eight notes of "The Colonel Bogey March."

5. You are fond of gizmos (defroster, minivacuum cleaner, travel shaver) that plug into the cigarette lighter.

6. You have a toy cat lying in the rear window whose eyes light up when you step on the brakes.

7. You have every road map in the glove compartment but the one you need.

8. You have a stereo system in the car that sounds better than the one in your house (and the one in the house isn't bad at all).

9. You have a change-holder or drink-holder attached to the dashboard, and you use both of them all the time.

10. You display any of the following bumper stickers:

a. "If you can read this, you're too damn close."

b. "I ❤ _____" (providing that the state loved is different from the one on the license plate).

c. "Have you hugged your child today?"

d. "Sailors have more fun" (providing the car is driven by someone who sailors have more fun than).

e. "I may be slow but I'm ahead of you."

f. "Love animals. Don't eat them."

g. "McGovern for president."

h. "55 saves lives" (providing the car is going 65 mph or more).

i. "Take it easy."

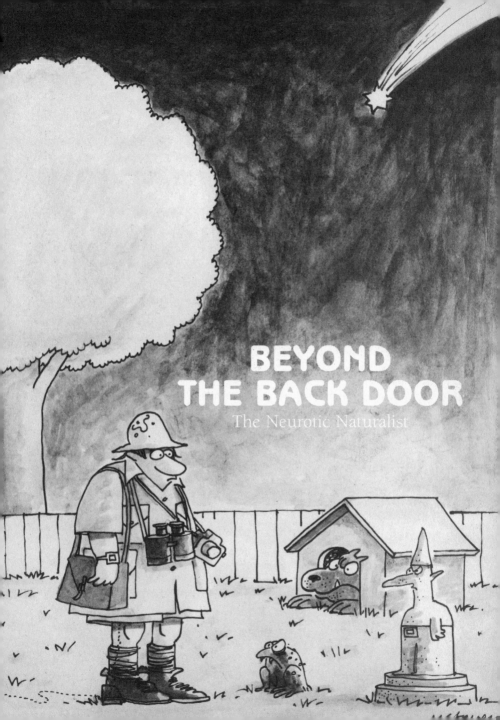

# BEYOND
# THE BACK DOOR
The Neurotic Naturalist

Unfortunately, at some point the neurotic must leave the comfort and safety of the home and go outdoors. This is a big step, but it really should be taken. There is no sense in maintaining, as some do, that nature can be observed perfectly well through the kitchen window or from the back seat of the car during a short drive. You can get away with a statement like that if you are Noel Coward or W. H. Auden, but most of us don't even speak with a British accent, so outdoors we must go.

We don't have to go rushing pell-mell into the deep woods, however. Those horrors can be put off a while longer. What we want to explore now is the world of the yard, the neighbor's yard, the neighborhood (or, if a city dweller, the park). These are the areas, familiar to us, where we believe we hold some control over things, where at the very least we are near enough to a telephone should nature begin to get the upper hand on us.

There is nothing quite like the feeling of dominion one experiences during a walk in the yard, the neighborhood, or the park on a pleasant day. Ideally, such walks should be conducted at a brisk pace so that only the benign surface aspects of nature are glimpsed. But often we are tempted to dawdle, to inspect, in short to look for trouble. Because of this curiosity—and because we wish to maintain our feeling of dominion—we should at all times make sure we are adequately prepared for these short hikes. Before setting out, we ought to be equipped with the following essentials:

**BUG REPELLENT.** This should be applied liberally, which is to say slathered on. Spray it all over your body before you put on your clothes. Spray it until it fizzes on your skin like butter on a hot skillet. Spray it on your clothes. Extra-heavy doses should be applied to your ears, neck, wrist, ankles, and the crooks of your elbows and knees, all of which mosquitoes find especially tender. It's a good idea to take some repellent along with you so you can quickly envelop yourself in a noxious cloud as the need arises.

**CLOTHES.** No one would suggest you wander naked through the neighborhood, of course, but a judicious choice of clothing can only enhance your pleasure. A long-sleeved turtleneck sweater whose neck you can pull up to cover your face would be good, as would thick kneesocks, industrial-strength denim pants, steel-toed boots, oven mitts, and a flap-eared biplane pilot's hat (with goggles).

**A CRUDE WALKING STICK OR STAFF.** This gives you a proprietary air as you walk, and it's also useful for fending off the yapping curs that race out from various yards along the way. A golf club (a three-iron is ideal) or a shillelagh will also make a convincing impression.

**A SHARP STICK FOR CURIOUS PROBING.** This is a good tool for poking at wasp nests, anthills, mole tunnels, tent caterpillar webs, tree warts, sprinkler heads, and assorted turds. Make sure this stick is sturdy yet long enough to assure you safe distance from the object under scrutiny.

**A KNIFE.** This can be used for cutting yourself free from clotheslines you might blunder into or tree roots you may unwittingly become ensnared in. A $700 Swiss Army knife or a good grape-fruit knife will do the job equally well.

**A FOLDING CHAIR.** You may come upon a beautiful but very slowly developing sunset, in which case you will want to be seated comfortably.

**A NOTEBOOK AND PENCIL.** These can be used for jotting down interesting bird sightings you may come across and also to mark down the license plate numbers of strange cars that seem to be prowling the neighborhood.

# A FEW HANDY TIPS

As we have indicated, the yard and neighborhood should prove to be a reasonably benign study area for neurotic naturalists. However, we must always remember that real discomfort and danger lie in wait even in the shadows of our own houses. Being properly equipped will help greatly, but there are also certain things we should keep in mind as we venture out:

1. Never stray far enough away from home that you can't run back without being out of breath. Let's say a yellow jacket starts chasing you. You don't want to be a mile or two away from home when that happens, because you will collapse in a heap far from the front door, and not only will the yellow jacket have its day, but your inert form will be likely be swarmed over by ants as well. A good rule of thumb is to stay close enough to home that you can hear the phone if it starts ringing.

2. Don't lie down barebacked on the lawn. No one knows why grass makes your back itch so much, but everyone knows that you won't be able to reach the spot that itches the most.

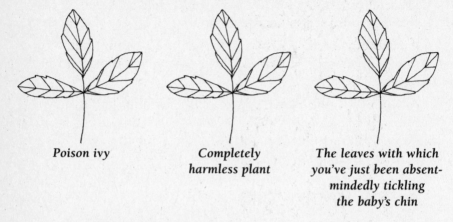

*Poison ivy*

*Completely
harmless plant*

*The leaves with which
you've just been absent-
mindedly tickling
the baby's chin*

3. A citronella candle will keep insects from landing on the candle. That is the extent of its effectiveness.

4. It is widely known that anyone who says, "I'm immune to poison ivy" is in for a bitter comeuppance. Experts claim that poison ivy can be contracted by touch, by breathing its smoke as it burns, by petting a dog that has been rolling in it, by walking close to it on a windy day, by dreaming about it with the windows open, and by mentioning its name while sipping a cool drink.

5. Always wait an hour or so after eating before going outdoors. Not doing so may result in a case of severe stomach cramps, and you may fall face down into a pile of leaves and suffocate.

6. If you allow a pricker bush to grow in your yard, you will live to regret it. Uproot it now.

## THE GRASS MENAGERIE

The vast area between the living room carpet and the forest primeval is covered mostly by people's lawns. Generally speaking, lawns are of more interest to psychologists than to naturalists; they harbor little in the way of interesting wildlife, yet their appearance often serves as a vivid reflection of their owners. And just as mountaineers often speak of "knowing" the mountain or voyageurs speak of "knowing" the river, so must the neighborhood neurotic get to "know" the neighbors. A great way to do this is through their lawns.

There are several basic types of lawns from which much can be learned:

**THE PLAYGROUND.** This is a scruffy hardscrabble patch scattered with hastily thrown-down bicycles, scooters, Hot Wheels, and other modes of juvenile transportation. This is the yard where all the neighborhood dogs congregate, where suspect lemonade is sold on hot summer days, and where a sweep of the balding turf will turn up everything from small plastic army men toting bazookas to many, many kitchen utensils correctly given up for lost long ago. Inside the house you can count on dirty soap in the soap dishes, fingermarks around all handles and knobs, and giant-sized loaves of soft white bread in the freezer. The playground is a very tough lawn on wildlife, although the house itself usually contains a lively assortment of natural creatures.

**THE ORNAMENTAL LAWN.** Perhaps a lawn jockey or a plaster drunk leaning against a plaster lamppost out front, perhaps a family of fake rabbits or a religious grotto out back. The ornamental lawn creates its own world (as we will see later on), a world that acknowledges nature but does not necessarily welcome it. Inside this house find bowls of candy, plenty of knickknacks, and perhaps a humorous toilet seat cover in the basement powder room.

**THE OBSESSIVE MANICURE JOB.** Here we find hedges that represent the highest expression of the topiary art, borders between lawn and sidewalk so straight they must have been worked out with a slide rule, and a lawn so soft, so full, so green that you want to have sex with it. Unfortunately, nature is strictly prohibited from entering such preserves, and any creature that accidentally wanders in will promptly be sprayed, zapped, or chased out. Nature is considered to be a dirty and unreliable intruder in the yard, and certainly indoors as well. Inside, find a haze of disinfectant, covers on the furniture, and a small dog that wears clothes.

**THE LAISSEZ-FAIRE LAWN.** Here is a lawn wildly overgrown and gone to weeds, very often located next door to the obsessive manicure job. This is the house with the snow shovel out on the front porch all year round and the hopelessly rusted barbecue grill out back. Nature thrives in this yard, using it as a home base for its forays out into the rest of the neighborhood. Indoors here, look for heavy-duty, Holiday Inn–type curtains on the bedroom windows and not much around the house for lunch.

# FAUNA ORNAMENTA

The inexperienced neighborhood neurotic is sometimes baffled by a species of brightly colored, rather rigid creatures that populate some yards, but not others. These aren't true natural creatures, though. They're lawn ornaments, and they have about as much to do with real life as root beer has to do with refined dining.

Nevertheless, many lawn ornament fanciers believe their statues play an important role in the natural world. They fuss over them, they converse with them, some even move them around the yard according to the time of day or herd them together on Christmas Eve. And so might we make use of them ourselves. Lawn ornament clusters make excellent practice zones for the budding naturalist. The plaster fauna are easy to sight and simple to sneak up on, and they are guaranteed to stand stock-still while we hone our note-taking skills on coloration and markings.

From time to time (especially in winter, when the activities of the true creatures in the neighborhood are sluggish), it might be a good idea to form a party and go out to observe the local lawn ornaments. Granted, they constitute a very weak link in the chain of life, but they *are* outdoors, and at least they look *something* like real animals.

We list here some of the more common members of the species:

**MOTHER DUCK AND DUCKLINGS.** Always seen in a line, with the mother duck in front and the baby ducks trailing behind. The lineup never varies because the overwhelming majority of people who own lawn ornaments do not fool around with them.

**PLASTER DEER.** Sometimes a delicate fawn, at other times a placid doe or a full-blown antlered buck. Sometimes momentarily mistaken for the real thing by passing motorists. Never mistaken for the real thing by passing deer, however.

**PINK FLAMINGOS.** Too weird for words, but quite thrilling as a quasi–nature sighting. Always seen in pairs, never in flocks.

**THE MEXICAN LEADING THE BURRO.** Rather large as lawn ornaments go, and rather mystifying as well. Were we not strictly concerned with nature, we might ask ourselves what the owner of such an ornament is trying to "say."

**THE MIRRORED BALL ON A PEDESTAL.** Although this item does not resemble an animal, it carries a totemic power that we cannot ignore. It is the ancient symbol of perfect harmony in the great outdoors (or perhaps a secret symbol designating the homes of unreconstructed Nazis). In any event, it wouldn't hurt to pray to it.

# THE FIELD GUIDE

Once we step from the house to the outdoors, we lose whatever claim we may have entertained regarding our mastery over nature. In the house, we presume that we have the upper hand. In the deep forest, it is nature that calls the shots. But in the yard or the neighborhood, we exist on an uneasy but equal footing with natural creatures: Sometimes we get them, sometimes they get us.

In short, it is in the yard that we can be regarded as simply another link in the ecosystem. We know who we are, but what of these others to whom we give up our blood, sweat, toil, and tears (and from whom we get very little in return)? A short field trip turns up the following:

## June Bug

**DESCRIPTION:** The closest thing to a flying beer can that nature offers.

**HABITAT:** June.

**HABITS:** Perhaps the clumsiest, noisiest creature in all the outdoors—a june bug simplemindedly going about its business on the porch in late spring can easily sound like a team of burglars trying to break down the front door. Likes to rattle around porch lights and repeatedly butt into windowpanes. Can often be found lying helplessly on its back, spinning in slow circles as its wings beat frantically. A disgrace to all other natural creatures.

**FOOD:** Never seems quite able to maneuver into position to eat.

**COMMENTS:** Those people who own and employ backyard bug zappers find great comfort in the steady cadence of *blips* and *zips* as minor insects fly into the coils. They should take note, however, that when a june bug hits a zapper it not only produces a horrifying *blaatt,* but it can also short-circuit the unit, destroy the zapper, and even knock out all electrical power for miles around.

## Gnat

**DESCRIPTION:** A small black flying insect hard to describe more properly because it is usually observed only after it has been fished out of the human eye, at which point it resembles a wet piece of black lint.

**HABITAT:** Likes to congregate in clouds around people's heads.

**HABITS:** The gnat's main purpose in life, evidently, is to gain entry into the human head at all costs. Whether this is accomplished through the eyes, nose, mouth, or ears doesn't seem to matter.

**FOOD:** Sweat, along with those unsavory tidbits found in eyes, ears, noses, and mouths.

**COMMENTS:** One theory regarding gnats is that they are attracted to the salt found in our eyes and in our sweat. An interesting experiment would be to go out and work up a good sweat on a hot day, then lie down on the ground with a bowl of salt next to your head. Do more gnats land on your face or in the bowl of salt? Try it.

## Mosquito

**DESCRIPTION:** A small winged messenger of evil, disease, and despair; the scum of life.

**HABITAT:** Anywhere that people are trying to relax and enjoy themselves.

**HABITS:** Spreads malaria, encephalitis, and yellow fever. Gets a kick out of swarming all over hapless picnickers, strollers, stargazers, and porch-sitters. Likes to buzz in and around people's ears, forcing them to slap themselves repeatedly on the side of the head.

**FOOD:** Blood, blood pudding, bloody Marys, etc.

**COMMENTS:** According to scientific reports, mosquitoes are growing more agile, more intelligent, and larger with each passing year. It is estimated that in about ten years they will be quicker than houseflies, a bit larger than crows, and as stealthy as Neapolitan pickpockets.

## The Neighbor's Dog

**DESCRIPTION:** A smelly, flea-infested hound with matted hair. A menace to the entire neighborhood.

**HABITAT:** Your yard.

**HABITS:** Likes digging frenetically in freshly planted flower beds, overturning your garbage can and strewing the embarrassing contents across the yard for all to see, chewing on the garden hose, baring its teeth malevolently at you whenever you venture out the door, barking all night at nothing, and crapping all over everything.

**FOOD:** Since its owners never feed it, this creature is perpetually crazed with hunger. Will eat anything, from yellow jackets to tulip bulbs to raw hotdogs (and then throw up somewhere on your property).

**COMMENTS:** The neighbor's dog has no understanding of even the most basic commands. It believes you are playing a new game when you order it to go home.

## Praying Mantis

**DESCRIPTION:** A pious green insect.

**HABITAT:** Found in the yards of truly good people, and also near churches.

**HABITS:** The praying mantis has turned its brief life over to helping mankind, the only insect to do so (so far). It is selfless, kind, dutiful, peaceful, and reverent. It tirelessly patrols lawns and gardens, looking for ways it can help the owners lead a more carefree life.

**FOOD:** It likes to eat insects that are harmful to people or injurious to people's pursuits.

**COMMENTS:** Praying mantises are protected by the law. If you are caught teasing one, you can be thrown into jail for a good long time. If you are caught killing one, you might be given the electric chair.

## Yellow Jacket

**DESCRIPTION:** A persistent, hot-tempered yellow hornet with a nasty sting.

**HABITAT:** Outdoor soft drink machines, punch bowls at outdoor wedding receptions, automobile dashboard areas.

**HABITS:** Likes to fly right at your face and then hover there, daring you to swat it away. Also likes to chase people for short distances around the yard (it knows by instinct which people are most likely to run). Will also lurk quietly under your car's dashboard until you have started the engine and begun driving; then it will suddenly fly at your face or land on the steering wheel and walk slowly toward your hands.

**FOOD:** Soft drinks. Will often crawl right into the bottle you are trying to drink from.

**COMMENTS:** "Don't bother it and it won't bother you" seems to be a saying expressly tailored for our relationship with yellow jackets. Too bad the yellow jackets don't know about it.

## Bat

**DESCRIPTION:** A scary winged animal with a criminal record as long as your arm.

**HABITAT:** Belfries, haunted houses, recurring nightmares.

**HABITS:** Enjoys flying dramatically in front of a full moon. Is attracted by long hair, in which it can be entangled for up to forty minutes (during which time it rabidly bites and claws at the head of the victim).

**FOOD:** Insects, virgin's blood.

**COMMENTS:** Actually, most bats are just harmless mammals that wish they were birds. In fact, they act just like birds, but they're so ugly (and they know it) that they confine their flying to the nighttime. Go out to observe them some night and you will see them hopping across the lawn, perching on signposts, hunting for worms, frolicking in the birdbath—doing all of the things that real birds do during the day. It's really sort of sad.

## Firefly

**DESCRIPTION:** A winged, easily captured insect; ostentatious, but endearingly so.

**HABITAT:** Hedges, the near woods, old jars with airholes punched into the lids.

**HABITS:** This totally benign creature exists solely for the momentary pleasure of small children. Its blinking signal says, "Here I am, kids!" They then capture the firefly and place it in a jar, where it blinks cheerfully until it dies of fatigue (about six hours after the kids get bored and move on to something else). Certainly, this is the hardest-working bug in show business.

**FOOD:** Odd bits of peanut butter, mayonnaise, jelly—whatever kind of jar it ends up in.

**COMMENTS:** Abraham Lincoln was so poor that even when he was living in the White House, he read at night by the light of fireflies that his beloved son Tad had captured along Pennsylvania Avenue.

# BAD BIRDS

Each year thousands of neurotic naturalists take up the absorbing hobby of bird watching or "birding" or "staring at trees." Thousands of others claim at cocktail parties that they have a keen interest in birds but are only making conversation. Still others claim to be bird-watchers only to justify the purchase of high-powered binoculars, which they put to more nefarious uses. And then there are millions who think of birds only as bony but tasty little morsels on a plate. For whatever reason, many people find it useful to be able to identify the birds they see (in the same way that others like to state proudly: "There goes a 1978 Buick"). This guide wishes to be of some help.

We are not interested in exotic species that no one, except for the truly crazed, ever sees. We don't care to differentiate between the calls of the long-billed dowitcher and the short-billed dowitcher, for instance, because we have never seen a dowitcher of any bill length and, besides, *dowitcher* sounds more like an obscure carpentry tool than a bird. We are far more interested in the birds that thrust themselves upon us, that fly heedlessly into picture windows, that squabble and bicker endlessly just outside the bedroom at 4:30 A.M., and that maliciously befoul the car windshield every chance they get. In short, we are interested in bad birds.

In order to identify even bad birds properly, it is first necessary to see them. It is therefore suggested that the bird-watcher spend quite a bit of money on ocular devices. These might include:

**EYEGLASSES.** If you suffer from very bad eyesight, it would be useless to venture outdoors without your glasses or contact lenses. You might think it intriguing to spot a circus clown dancing high in an oak tree, but such blurred images do not advance your knowledge of bird life. Bring your specs.

**MONOCLE.** This eyepiece gives you a jaunty air but is more suited to the drawing room than to the great outdoors. Lorgnettes, microscopes, magnifying glasses, and jeweler's loupes are also unsuitable for birding and are best left at home.

**KALEIDOSCOPE.** This is a good item to bring along in case the bird watching gets dull (as it always does). Paint the outside of the tube black so others will think you are seriously scanning the treetops.

**BINOCULARS.** If you think you've got a steady hand, just wait until you try to discern the shape of a bird's beak from five hundred yards through a pair of powerful binoculars. In less than thirty seconds you'll feel like a terminal case in a detox ward. Much better to rest the binoculars on a windowsill and look in on the neighbors (and don't forget to turn out the lights in your viewing room).

**TELESCOPE.** For the serious birder. Not to be confused with the spyglass, which is for the serious pirate.

**ELECTRON TELESCOPE.** For the very serious birder who wishes to view bird life on Saturn or the Andromeda constellation as well as in the neighborhood. Sure to impress your companions.

Once you have obtained your viewing devices, it will be time to begin birding. This can be done either by going out on a field trip or by merely tossing some stale bread or suet out the door and then watching by a window as the squirrels come flocking. Generally speaking, the nicer birds appear in other people's yards while you get only the squirrels and an occasional starling or crow. Because self-deception is an important aspect of bird watching, however, it won't be long before your notebook is brimming with unlikely sightings. Be that as it may, here's a brief guide to the birds that actually show up—the bad birds.

# Crow

**DESCRIPTION:** A large black flying garbage disposal; rather over-bearing in close company. There is no such thing as a female crow. Or a male crow. Crows have only one sex: crow.

**VOICE:** Broderick Crawford at seventy-eight rpms. Rarely has a nice thing to say about anyone or anything.

**HABITAT:** Enjoys loitering boldly at the sides of busy highways, cursing the passing traffic. Also likes to mass together ominously after dark in huge treetop social groups.

**BAD HABITS:** By day, the crow menaces farmers and their crops for a few hours and then flies off to feed on fast-food french fries carelessly tossed away by motorists. By night, gathering with thousands of pals, the crow plays cards, smokes cheap cigars it has found during the day, and swaps filthy stories until dawn.

**COMMENTS:** The crow may well become the first bird bold enough to come right into the house, pistol-whip the residents, get what it wants, and then fly out again.

# Pigeon

**DESCRIPTION:** An overweight urban dove with an iridescent neck and funky little head movements much imitated by dancing humans.

**VOICE:** A faint burbling coo. If you can hear it, it means the pigeon is probably close enough to be flecking your window ledge with disease-ridden droppings.

**HABITAT:** Cities the world over. Within the cities, pigeons particularly enjoy marring churches, banks, and other distinguished buildings with ornate facades.

**BAD HABITS:** The pigeon has much in common with the house-fly: It feeds on the most disgusting filth imaginable, it spreads disease, and when alarmed it flies away, only to return moments later to the exact same spot. Befriends unstable people just to get food from them. Ridicules the accomplishments of our illustrious forefathers by fecklessly perching on the heads of statues. Likes to appear on national TV by landing on baseball and football fields while a game is in progress.

**COMMENTS:** If you wish to experience a nameless terror, look into the eyes of a pigeon.

## Blue Jay

**DESCRIPTION:** Proof that looks aren't everything. A handsome blue-crested bird with sharp features and a testy temperament.

**VOICE:** A shrill, insistent shriek with all the charm of a dentist's drill, or, at rare, quieter moments, a pathetic wheedling.

**HABITAT:** A bully at heart, the blue jay hides during the summer, when there are a lot of birds its size around, then emerges during the winter, when the only birds left are chickadees and juncos and wrens—all birds the blue jay can easily boss around.

**BAD HABITS:** Likes to chase small starving birds away from feeders. Will sometimes sneak into the nests of other birds and either eat the eggs it finds there, maliciously destroy them, or just vandalize the nests for kicks. Enjoy pecking the eyes out of children's dolls accidentally left out in the yard.

**COMMENTS:** Blue jays can be intimidated and silenced by the presence of massed crows, but bringing in crows to silence blue jays would be like hiring a drummer to block out the sound of a leaky faucet.

## Seagull

**DESCRIPTION:** A large white-and-gray bird with a serious problem.

**VOICE:** A piercing cry that when heard in the distance can be very pleasant and nostalgic, but when heard nearby or directly overhead can be maddening.

**HABITAT:** Used to be content with a simple life by the sea.

Recently, however, this once noble bird has fallen into league with crows, pigeons, and other miscreants as a lover of garbage. It's now quite commonly seen flocking greedily around huge urban garbage dumps. This is a bird on a bender.

**BAD HABITS:** Hovers around the wakes of seagoing vessels, eagerly diving after bread crusts, bottle caps, film wrappers, discarded jokers from decks of cards, and anything else thrown overboard. Kills helpless clams and mussels by dropping them from great heights onto rocks or concrete pavement. Likes to ride on garbage scows and plunge its beak into the fresh, steaming garbage it finds there, completely oblivious to the spectacle it is making of itself.

**COMMENTS:** The seagull's complete loss of self-respect in recent years is a classic symptom of the addictive personality. Its obsessive craving for garbage should be seen as an illness rather than as a crime. Gull Outreach Centers are being formed, but funds are short. You can help—or you can turn the page.

## Mockingbird

**DESCRIPTION:** A slim, lizardy-looking bird with a big mouth, a bag of tired vaudeville turns, and the entertainment value of a third-rate magician at an Elks Club smoker.

**VOICE:** Unrelenting.

**HABITAT:** Likes to find the most prominent perch available and then work from there. Ideally would like to score a big contract with a major Las Vegas revue.

**BAD HABITS:** Will seemingly do anything to attract attention, like Mickey Rooney or Sammy Davis, Jr., at their worst. Will reward even the briefest malevolent glance with an extra two hours of patter.

**COMMENT:** Vaudeville is dead.

# THE GARDEN

As the animals of the great African plains congregate at water holes, so do the creatures of the neighborhood and the near woods gather at vegetable gardens. And why shouldn't they? Gardens provide them with a great variety of fresh produce, including many items they would otherwise never think of adding to their diets. Gardens offer a plush, loamy dining environment. And, finally, gardens are continually nurtured and replenished by the thoughtful, hardworking gardening staff. For natural creatures this amounts to breakfast in bed every day at a swank hotel, and they would be foolish to shy away from it.

It is therefore a good idea for the neurotic naturalist to plant a vegetable garden. In doing so, you are summoning the natural world to your own yard; you are announcing that yours is a place of peace and bounty. Planting a garden is the suburban or country equivalent of feeding the pigeons. It will make you feel good, and it will make the animals feel very, very good.

To make sure that a wide sampling of creatures visits your garden, you might consider doing the following:

**USE NATURAL FERTILIZER.** A sad fact of nature is that animals are attracted to manure—their own, that of their colleagues in the same species, indeed manure in general holds for them a fascination that we, thankfully, have evolved beyond. Lay down a carpet of fresh fertilizer and not only will all sorts of animals come sniffing curiously, but the food you have planted for them will grow more strongly and abundantly.

**WATER THE GARDEN REGULARLY.** During the dry summer months, natural creatures become thirsty, dusty, and cranky. While slugs will drink beer, most animals prefer water, which you can give them by soaking your garden from time to time.

And if you are really generous with the water, you may want to stock your garden with trout and go fishing there during the long lazy days between planting and harvesting.

**PLANT CORN.** This crop, though relatively difficult to grow, is a surefire way of attracting truly exotic fauna into your yard. Not only do insects greatly appreciate this vegetable, but crows, raccoons, opossums, deer, bears, moose, and just plain hungry passersby enjoy a plump ear fresh off the stalk.

**ERECT A FENCE.** The act of building a fence around the garden will give the animals that feed there a sense of belonging. They will consider your garden to be "their special place," now made off-limits to would-be interlopers. And you may find pleasure in your new dual roles as gardener and zookeeper.

# "DO YOU FEEL OKAY? YOU LOOK PALE"

Health and Health Care for the Neurotic

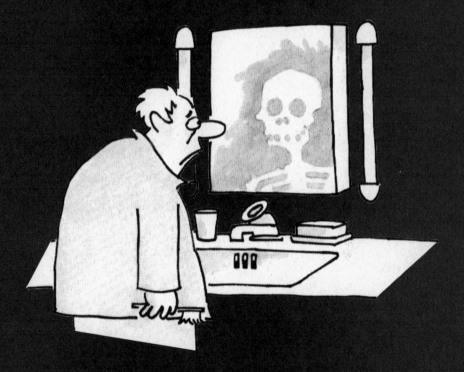

# THE BIG PICTURE

Every chest pain is a heart attack; every headache is a brain tumor. You tell people about the heart attack, but you keep the brain tumor to yourself—it will be fatal, after all, and there's nothing that anyone can do.

This is the basic approach to health and health care for the neurotic. Not only can you expect the worst, but the worst actually is happening to you right now. When Alexander Pope wrote, "Here am I, dying of a hundred good symptoms," he was expressing the essential neurotic theme (except that he really was dying). The true neurotic would have added, "And no one seems to realize it."

The neurotic operates in a perpetual twilight of ill health that is dimmed further by confusing magazine articles, know-nothing specialists who picked up their medical degrees in Central America, and hundreds of colorfully packaged health products that just don't do the job. He or she is a walking catalogue of ailments and complaints in a body that is as finely tuned as the most exquisite and temperamental motorcar; if any one small thing goes wrong, it easily can lead to a breakdown of the entire machine.

Certain ailments, however, are particularly well suited to the neurotic:

On the lowest level are the minor bruises (caused by shopping carts, coffee tables, unrestrained dancing partners) that must be probed with the fingers, and the muscle strains and aches that must be kneaded and flexed until one feels the reassuring stab of pain. When in company, one should emphasize each flex with a brief, badly hidden wince; the injury itself should always be referred to as a "ligament pull" and accompanied by a lie ("I was mountain climbing," "I was mobbed at the airport"). In this same category there are also the cuts, scrapes, and careless gashes that must be attended to with ointments and bandages. These injuries (referred to as "abrasions" or "lacerations") should frequently be peeked at under the bandages for signs of infection lest gangrene set in and amputation be deemed necessary.

On a somewhat higher plane of worry are the rashes and fungal growths. These are good if they appear suddenly and without explanation, and more wonderful yet if they don't itch. "I've got this damn rash and I don't know where it came from. Look," might be a neurotic's sly gambit at a cocktail party. Such a procedure is not recommended for fungal growths, however, since they usually are located in embarrassing spots and no one (not even doctors) wants to see them.

The next level is the neurotic's specialty—disorienting ailments. These are valued because they may be called in to explain spells of unusual behavior that are in reality of a strictly mental nature. Hypoglycemia, or low blood sugar, is the current leader of the pack here, although inner-ear ailments, sinus conditions, and allergies remain useful, too. Each of these ailments can be signaled by dizziness, lethargy, and jumpiness—all hallmarks of the anxiety attack. Such symptoms are nonspecific enough that one can go to the doctor and simply say, "I feel kind of funny all over" or "I feel like a bird in a cage." Doctors love to hear this.

Finally, there are the major illnesses, or rather the fear of major illnesses. The fear is constant and wide-ranging; it usually is triggered by some minor occurrence that, in the neurotic's beehive mind, indicates big trouble ahead. This phenomenon might best be shown by the following chart:

| *Symptom* | *Probable cause* |
| --- | --- |
| cough | lung cancer |
| bloody nose | brain hemorrhage |
| blurry vision | incipient blindness |
| sneeze | pneumonia |
| pain in side | appendicitis |
| twitching eyelid | stroke |
| rash | syphilis |
| headache | brain tumor |
| lethargy | leukemia |
| stomachache | botulism |
| pain in arm | heart attack |

## THE UNHAPPY ORGAN

Recently it has become fashionable for one to develop more of an awareness of one's body, to become more closely acquainted with what it is, what parts are contained by it, and how it all works. This is nothing new for neurotics. Not only are they already acquainted with their bodies, but they have been on fairly intimate speaking terms with them for years. During that time (despite the rather one-sided nature of these conversations) a certain familiarity has set in; indeed, in some cases this familiarity has reached the point where important organs seem to have acquired shapes and personalities that are alarmingly Disneyesque.

The neurotic's relationship with his or her body is a peculiar one anyway. It is founded not on any notion of harmony but rather on the assumption that each organ is a potential killer and that it will kill if given the slightest opportunity to do so. It is a relationship based on fear and false information, the result of which is an interior landscape that is strange and wondrous to behold:

## Brain
**APPEARANCE:** Gray, jellyish mound with ridges. Damp yet somehow electrified. Secret passageways, forgotten regions, frightening depths, disappointing shallows.
**FUNCTION:** Key. Runs the show.
**DANGERS:** Air bubbles from careless inoculations, destruction from alcoholic beverages (two beers = 600,000 brain cells), religious cults, junk on television, LSD, comic books, small-town life, filing and collating.

## Heart
**APPEARANCE:** Not heart-shaped. Pulsating, occasionally palpitating, looks something like bagpipes. Blood all over the place.
**FUNCTION:** Pumps blood, prompts irrational decisions, fosters true love.
**DANGERS:** Four-egg omelets, love from afar, the Chicago Cubs, phone calls at 3 A.M., telegrams, monsters.

## Liver
**APPEARANCE:** Surprisingly large, slick brown slab. Extremely nondescript.
**FUNCTION:** Secretes bile, produces liver spots; seat of desire.

**DANGERS:** Serious, steady boozing, dirty inoculation needles, airplane glue.

## Kidneys
**APPEARANCE:** Two of them, very moist. Shaped like swimming pools.
**FUNCTION:** Clean blood, dry it, iron it, put it away.
**DANGERS:** Driving a taxi or a bus, kidney punches from overenthusiastic uncles, hat pins, kidney stones (the worst pain there is).

## Lungs
**APPEARANCE:** Two bellowslike items. Can be pink, brown, black.
**FUNCTION:** Air comes in, air goes out.
**DANGERS:** Cigarettes without filters, cigarettes with filters, something that "goes down the wrong pipe," being stuck in traffic behind a bus, "sucking" wounds, textile dust, anything to do with coal.

## Stomach
**APPEARANCE:** Never quite what it should be.
**FUNCTION:** Holds food (usually); rates blind dates.
**DANGERS:** Thanksgiving, bayonet warfare, swimming right after eating, miracle diets, a doubleheader at the ballpark, rollercoasters.

## Bladder
**APPEARANCE:** Rubbery bag, much more strongly developed in women.
**FUNCTION:** Holds urine, but not indefinitely.
**DANGERS:** Long movies at which you are seated in the middle of a crowded row, long car rides on bumpy roads with a sadistic

driver who won't pull over and stop, long anything, beerfests, tickling.

## Appendix
**APPEARANCE:** Seemingly harmless sliver.
**FUNCTION:** Causes pain, sometimes death.
**DANGERS:** Camping in remote areas, unforeseen complications during its removal.

## Intestines
**APPEARANCE:** Large and small coiled tubes, actually over seven hundred miles long.
**FUNCTION:** Conductor of the Bowel Movement.
**DANGERS:** Tapeworms, swallowing coins or campaign buttons, bizarre jungle fevers, mysterious obstructions, drinking from water holes that are surrounded by sun-bleached cattle skulls.

# TEN UNIVERSAL TIPS REGARDING HEALTH AND SAFETY

1. Someday you'll cross your eyes and they'll *stay* crossed.

2. Many, many people have bled to death by inexpertly trying to remove their own warts. Don't try it.

3. Every athletic coach is personally acquainted with at least one youngster who was blinded by someone snapping a wet towel in the locker room. Don't do it.

4. You can get cancer just from being pinched on the arm.

5. Any time you get hit in the temple by anything, forget it. The temple is the A-1 death zone on the human body. Once there was this guy who was mowing his lawn with a power

mower when he ran over a tiny pebble that shot fifty yards across the street and hit an innocent boy in the temple. The boy died without even getting a chance to whimper. That's how dangerous the temple is.

6. The only thing that can challenge the temple is the Triangle of Death that comes on the top of every newborn baby's head. Don't touch it. Don't ask questions, just don't touch it.

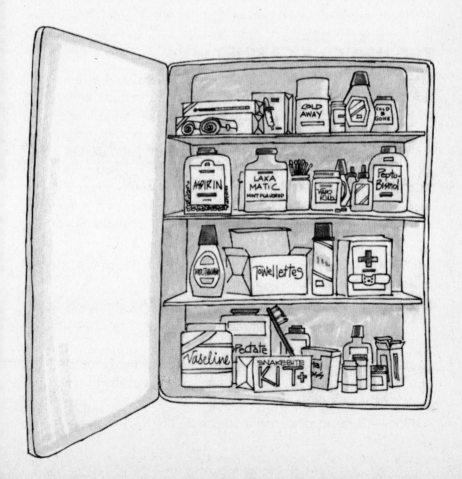

7. Spiders are attracted to heavily lacquered bouffant hairdos. They live there and eat their way into the skull.

8. The centers of golf balls are filled with deadly acid that can easily squirt into your eyes if you happen to smash a ball with a hammer.

9. Don't put coins in your mouth. You don't know where they've been.

10. Don't sit down on a toilet seat at a gas station.

## THE MEDICINE CABINET

When things are not going well, the medicine cabinet is often the place to turn to. A well-stocked cabinet will almost always offer something that you can take that will make you feel better (even if there is nothing wrong with you). The properly maintained medicine cabinet should contain at least the following:

**ACE BANDAGES—(2 SIZES)** Worn for minor strains; especially useful to wear when someone wants you to help paint a house. Also, they attract attention and lead to conversations about health.

**THERMOMETERS—(2)** Second one was bought when the first seemed to be stuck at 98.6 degrees.

**EAR SYRINGE—**For removal of ear wax. Used once, improperly, as water ended up streaming down the side of your face and shoulder and onto the floor.

**COLD REMEDIES—(6)** Capsules, pills, liquids. All used especially *in anticipation* of a cold. Do not operate farm machinery while under the influence of these remedies.

**ASPIRIN—**Gigantic, department store–size bottle. Always try to shake out just two tablets into your hand, as they do in the commercials.

**LAXATIVE**—Mint flavored.

**Q-TIPS**—For minor, curious probing. Be careful not to puncture your eardrum. Bury them deep in the wastebasket after using them; they are not something that anyone else particularly wants to see.

**VICKS VAPORUB**—Wonderful fumes make you sob and ask for Mommy.

**EYEDROPS**—For redness. Two drops in each eye and seven or eight on your cheeks and eyebrows.

**NOSE DROPS**—Highest strength, to prevent accidental suffocation while sleeping.

**PEPTO-BISMOL**—To be taken once chest pains are determined not to be a heart attack. Pleasing minty taste.

**MOUTHWASH**—Get the one that tastes the best, maybe a fresh mint flavor.

**MOIST TOWELETTES**—Good for anxiety attacks.

**BACTINE AND BAND-AIDS**—For lavish care of little scrapes and booboos.

**VASELINE**—No medicine cabinet is complete without it.

**KAOPECTATE**—If you have to use it, it's already too late.

**SNAKEBITE KIT**—You never know. Instructions make for fascinating toilet reading.

**MYSTERIOUS TOOTHBRUSH**—Not yours because you would never buy that color.

**DENTAL FLOSS**—Waxed, mint flavored.

**PRESCRIPTIONS**—Tightly capped amber vials with pithy directions and your name misspelled. Soldiers under your command in the struggle against infirmity:

1. Knockout pills
2. Mood enhancers
3. Real cough syrup
4. Going-outside pills
5. Staying-inside pills
6. Breathing pills
7. Earache drops from six years ago
8. Yellow pills with missing label
9. An empty vial

## THE NEUROTIC'S TOP TEN REMEDIES

There are certain products that cannot properly be called medicine but which nevertheless offer endless comfort to the hypochondriac. These items are more likely to be found on the neurotic's person than in a medicine cabinet because one is never sure when the relief they offer will be needed. The key common denominator among these products is that they can be used freely whenever the urge is felt—there is no limit to how many or how much you can administer to yourself. This means that there is no real medicine involved here, but it is the ritual that is important; the *sense* of well-being is all.

1. **PINE BROTHERS COUGH DROPS.** Any of the popular cough drops can be included here, but Pine Brothers stand out because they are the only remedies that are almost exactly like Jujubes.

2. **SUCRETS.** For the tin box, the little tinfoil wrappers, and the pleasing, slightly numbing sensation on the tongue.

3. **CLORETS.** Nice green color. Green cross on the box has a gratifyingly antiseptic ring.

4. **ASPERGUM.** Perfect for neurotics whose throats contract to the size of keyholes at the thought of swallowing a whole aspirin tablet.

5. **TUMS.** Can anything that is "for the tummy" be considered serious medicine?

6. **DENTYNE.** The pieces are so small that they *must* be good for you.

7. **VICKS INHALER.** For the extremely nose conscious. Something you can be sure no one will ask to borrow.

8. **BENGAY.** The balm for troubled, twitching muscles. The heat and the vapors are inordinately pleasing.

9. **CHAPSTICK.** At least three flavors should always be on hand and in constant use.

10. **DR. BRONNER'S PEPPERMINT OIL PURE-CASTILE SOAP.** Shampoo with it, bathe, brush your teeth, cure athlete's foot, wash the car, fix the television, get your breakfast, you name it. The neurotic's great all-purpose product.

## TETANUS QUESTIONS

You've just cut your finger on a rusty nail. When was your last tetanus shot? Are you sure? How long are they good for? Why do you always get a different answer whenever you ask anyone? Are the shots good for that period of time no matter how many times you cut yourself on a rusty nail? Are you sure?

# THE VITAMIN GUIDE

Everyone is worried about vitamins, and rightly so. They are important to good health but they are very small and hard to see, so you never can be sure just which ones and how many of them you are getting in a normal meal. You hope for the best, of course, but hope alone is not enough to ward off scurvy, rickets, and keratomalacia.

In this regard we must all face the questions of the minimum daily requirement. First of all, what is it? What does *minimum* mean in this context—minimum for good health or minimum just to stay alive? How many days in a row can you go without meeting it before you become comatose? Is there a maximum? What happens if you exceed it? Do you burst? (Recently the "minimum daily requirement" was changed to the "recommended daily allowance." Why? What the hell does *allowance* mean? Who's behind this thing?)

These are questions to face but not necessarily answer. Easier to explain is the role each vitamin plays in our lives and what specific problems we can expect if we do not meet our allowances of each.

**VITAMIN A.** Found most abundantly in liver. Deficiency causes night blindness. If you have any trouble seeing things in the dark, you might check out your vitamin A intake before it's too late.

**VITAMINS B1, B2, B6, B12, B24, B48, ETC.** The B team can be found most reliably in liver. Deficiencies here can lead to pernicious anemia, lip lesions, difficulty in breathing, seizures, and sluggish elimination. If all these occur at once, be sure to close the bathroom door, particularly if there are guests in the house.

**VITAMIN C.** Commonly to be found in the livers of grapefruit and oranges. This is the vitamin often used by unscrupulous purveyors of junk food and drink to give their products a healthful gloss. Deficiency can lead to spongy gums and the singing of bawdy sea chanteys.

**VITAMIN D.** Found in good quantity in fish-liver oil. "Big-boned" young women and men for whom dieting seems worthless might note that a deficiency of vitamin D can often lead to osteoporosis, a bone-thinning disease.

**VITAMIN E.** Found in encouraging volume in beef liver, this vitamin has been run through the mill in recent years. Next to the equally disappointing musk oil, vitamin E was touted as the great aphrodisiac of the 1970s. It enjoyed a brief flowering but now has fallen back on the list with rhinoceros powder and other bits and pieces of endangered species. Deficiency here can cause impotence, pallor, and grave doubt.

**VITAMIN H.** Also known as biotin, this vitamin is more frequently than not to be found in liver. Deficiencies here can produce limb paralysis, balding, and graying fur. At least that's what happened to the cuddly little animals that were cruelly taken out of their natural habitats and tortured on laboratory operating tables.

**VITAMIN K.** Found in fishmeal. Lack of it can lead to unchecked bleeding. Be sure never to run with the scissors in your hand if you haven't been eating your fishmeal.

# FIRST AID

Neurotics hate to be put on the spot, and they certainly do not like to be thrust into positions of responsibility during major medical emergencies, but occasionally they have no choice. Sometimes there is no one with a cool head around to take charge, and the neurotic is called upon to fill the breach. If your friend is dying, after all, you don't just stand there wringing your hands and humming an indistinct tune.

You have to rise to the occasion, and in order to do that you have to be prepared. In order to be prepared you should memorize the following instructions.

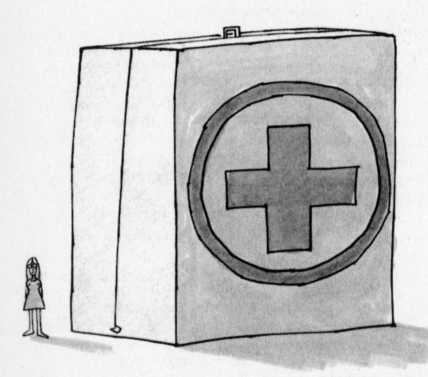

## Snakebites

1. Don't let the snake bite you, too. Hide behind a tree until the snake slithers off.

2. If the snake lingers in the area, throw rocks and sticks at it from a safe distance (thirty to forty feet).

3. Once you reach the victim, apply a tourniquet above the bite. You can use a belt or a tie for the tourniquet, although the chances that a person in the vicinity of an attacking snake will be wearing a tie are very slim.

4. Scream for help.

5. Suck the venom out of the wound. This sounds disgusting (and it is), but the bitter taste can be masked if you fill your mouth with applesauce before applying your lips to the fang marks.

6. Loosen the tourniquet. Look around to see if the snake has come back. Tighten the tourniquet. Suck on the wound again.

7. Tell the victim that everything's going to be okay.

8. Take the victim to the hospital.

9. Never go back to that place again.

## Conniption Fits

1. If the victim is pounding his head against the wall, grab him and fling him to the ground.

2. Pin the victim's arms and legs to the ground.

3. Say, "This is going to hurt me more than it's going to hurt you."

4. Slug the victim.

5. Take the victim's wallet out of his pocket and place it between your teeth to prevent yourself from screaming on account of pain from your broken hand.

6. Take yourself to the hospital. (And a job well done.)

## Electric Shock

1. Do not touch the person if he still is twitching, unless you want to get electrocuted yourself.

2. Turn off all the electricity.

3. Quickly run next door to borrow a flashlight from your neighbor.

4. Relocate victim. Probe him with a *dry* stick or an ax with a wooden handle to see if he still is alive.

5. If not dead, keep warm. If dead, apply ice.

6. Send for an ambulance and an electrician.

## Swallowed Foreign Bodies

1. Rounded objects such as marbles, buttons, silver dollars, golf balls, and duckpin bowling balls usually pass right through the intestinal tract. Simply regard the stool at a safe distance through binoculars every day until you have noted the passage of the object.

2. Oddly shaped objects such as open safety pins, nails, razor blades, and certain English hard candies may cause trouble, but usually not. Follow procedure for rounded objects unless victim stops breathing. If victim stops breathing, it means he is dead. Call undertaker.

3. Do not force-feed laxatives to the victim.

4. Do not turn the victim upside down and shake him.

5. Do not attempt an amateur tracheotomy on the victim.

6. Try not to make the victim feel like a jerk.

## Frostbite

1. Book a seat on the next flight to Florida.

2. Warm the victim gradually to 140 degrees.

3. Peel off the frostbitten parts *carefully* with a Swiss Army knife.

4. Take a nip or two of brandy.

5. Apply dressing to the raw, open wounds. French or Russian is good; Roquefort is extra. Do *not* apply oil and vinegar.

6. Take a little more brandy. Pour some over the victim.

7. Eat the victim.

## Hiccups

1. Laugh good-naturedly at the victim's predicament for several minutes.

2. Tell victim you have to go to the bathroom.

3. Sneak back into the room wearing a gorilla suit.

4. Suddenly leap out in front of the victim, screaming in his face.

5. Pause to see if hiccups persist.

6. If they do, force the victim to chug a half-gallon of tap water while standing on his head.

7. If all else fails, either have victim place his finger in a light socket or place your hands over his mouth and nose until he collapses from lack of air. (A pillow may also be used to smother the victim.)

## Radiation Exposure

1. Get the hell out of the area.
2. Wash all parts of your body with soap and water. Wash over and over again for seven months.
3. Burn everything you own.
4. Contact the local authorities for further instructions.
5. If the local authorities are all dead, contact enemy authorities or God.
6. If the local authorities are pretending that nothing untoward has happened, place a No Nukes bumper sticker on your car and make an appointment to see your doctor in thirty years.

## Stab Wounds

1. If the assailant still is armed with a knife or ice pick, try to appeal to his sense of decency and get him to drop the weapon.
2. If the assailant is armed with an ax or a chain saw, do *not* attempt to reason with him. Play dead, if possible.
3. Once the assailant has fled, go over and ask the victim who the first president of the United States was. This is to check if his faculties are intact.
4. If he says George Washington or even Alexander Hamilton

or Lyndon Johnson, he is on the right track and okay (though perhaps a bit stupid). If he says something ridiculous, such as Nellie Melba or Whirlaway, he doesn't have much time left.

5. Move the victim to a rain-slicked pavement underneath a lone streetlight.

6. Call in the victim's mother, an Irish Catholic priest, and a harmonica player.

7. Maintain a hushed reverence as the victim delivers a poignant soliloquy and then dies in his mother's arms.

# "I CAN'T BREATHE"

## The Neurotic Looks for Love

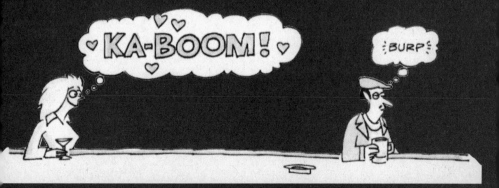

You feel faint. Your pulse is racing. You are haunted by a feeling of insecurity that does not seem justified. You are unable to concentrate on anything for more than a minute or two; you are unable to make any sense of what people are saying to you. The question is: Are you in love, or are you merely having another anxiety attack?

There are two reasons why this is not an easy question to answer:

1. Neurotics fall in love two or three times a month.
2. Anyone who is in love is neurotic.

Neurotics believe in a flawless, ideal sort of love, at least until they get married. They are prone to crushes. The objects of their ardor often are far away or married to a friend or on the cover of *People* magazine or otherwise unattainable. This unavailability makes neurotics feel very happy and very sad at the same time, a feeling that physically is almost exactly the same as the one you get when you are in an airplane flying through heavy turbulence. But instead of calling themselves "sick" and going to see a doctor, neurotics call themselves "romantic" and go to see an astrologer.

Although many neurotics sit around at home expecting love to come knocking at the front door, this very rarely happens. Eventually we have to snap out of our rich and extraordinarily fulfilling fantasy lives; we have to go out and take a look around. This "looking around" can be unpleasant business, and it means that we have to get involved in a lot that has nothing at all to do with true love. It means such things as going roller-skating for the first time and laughing whenever we fall down, or cavalierly pretending that it doesn't matter when a scoop of ice cream falls out of the cone and onto the seat of the car. It means dating. And dating almost always means trouble.

## THE DATING GAME

Neurotics usually fall in love with someone first, and then start dating, and then fall out of love. Occasionally they can get away without ever going out with the person they are in love with, and sometimes they can manage not even to talk to the person (thus preserving the love in its purest state), but more often than not a date is set and, over the course of an evening, the petty disappointments reveal themselves.

And how could they *not* reveal themselves, given the neurotic's strict standards? A piece of spinach caught in the teeth of a date spells doom. A mispronounced word here, a print on the wall of dogs playing poker there, and the whole arrangement is shot. The truth is, while neurotics are willing to overlook major character flaws (a lengthy record of armed robbery convictions, a penchant for dozing off at the wheel of the car), they demand nothing less than perfection in the little things of life. And perfection, in this context, means agreement.

Dating a neurotic can be a harrowing experience, not so much for anything that happens during the date itself as for the inexplicable silences that follow. The date is left wondering what went wrong, but the neurotic knows. The neurotic has been watching, and quietly checking off flaws. Here are a few of the danger signals that can convince a neurotic that Things Just Aren't Going to Work Out.

## On a Dinner Date
1. Your date attempts to be clever with the waiter—and fails.
2. A strolling violinist comes over and plays as if you were deeply in love when actually it is your first date together.
3. Your date holds the eating utensils like a prison inmate.
4. Your date doesn't finish dinner and then orders a huge dessert and finishes it all.
5. Your date goes into the kitchen to personally congratulate the chef for what you thought was a mediocre dinner.
6. Your date loudly joins in on the singing of "Happy Birthday" for celebrants at a nearby table.

## On a Dancing Date
1. Your date insists on doing the limbo.
2. Your date is completely drenched in sweat after two dances.
3. Your date yells inappropriate requests to the band.
4. Your date is a much better dancer than you are and you both know it.
5. Your date seriously injures a stranger on the dance floor with a flying elbow.
6. Your date does a modern interpretive dance to a Jerry Lee Lewis song.

## On a Movie, Play, or Concert Date

1. Your date tries to prove he or she knows when the music ends by starting to applaud just before it does.

2. Your date sprawls in an unseemly way.

3. Your date loudly discusses abortion politics while standing in line in front of the theater.

4. You notice that your (male) date's thighs are skinnier than yours are.

5. Your date spends half the play trying to read the *Playbill* in the dark.

6. Your date answers rhetorical questions that are posed on stage.

## On a Bar Date

1. Your date seems to be flirting with the bartender.

2. Your date goes to the bathroom and doesn't come out for twenty-three minutes.

3. Your date becomes sullen after one drink.

4. Your date starts lighting matches just for fun.

5. Your date absolutely insists on a certain brand of gin.

6. Your date asks people at neighboring tables for the cherries in their drinks.

## The Blind Date

The blind date was first practiced in the Dark Ages when the chieftains of barbarian tribes used to torture captured spies by fixing them up with disastrous dates until the spies gave in and revealed all they knew. Like the cockroach, the blind date has remained essentially unaffected by the passage of time. Today, in its most prevalent form, the blind date is a device used by happily married couples to torture their single friends just for the sake of a few laughs.

Because neurotics fear the unknown above all else, they find blind dating to be an appalling exercise to which they will consent only when they either are drunk or have had a few too many drinks. After all, who wants to take a chance like that? Who needs the humiliation? Who says I'm that desperate? On the other hand, you never know.

Here are a few tips to remember when you've sobered up:

1. **EXPECT THE WORST.** Your partner for the evening has been described as being "nice" or "cute" or "successful" or "recently divorced." Don't believe any of it except for the "recently divorced" part. You are not about to latch onto a prize. Other people latch onto prizes. If you expect the worst, anything above rock bottom will be a bonus.

2. **LOOKS AREN'T EVERYTHING.** You've been told this all your life, and you've even said it to yourself a few times. Here's another chance to put your goodness on the line, even though you certainly understand that looks *do help* in a situation such as this.

3. **QUICKLY ESTABLISH THE OTHER PERSON AS THE "BLIND DATE."** You will probably be accompanied by the couple who set up the date in the first place. Talk to them, laugh with them, throw in a couple of references that your date couldn't possibly understand. Do everything you can to establish yourself as being "closer" to the sponsors. Dominate the proceedings.

4. **YOU ARE NOT RESPONSIBLE FOR ANYTHING THAT GOES WRONG.** The date wasn't your idea, so you needn't feel

responsible for the conduct of the chef, the band, the movie projectionist, or random strangers you happen to pass on the sidewalk—as you would on a normal date. You might even be able to have fun.

5. **SOME THINGS NOT TO DO.** Don't bring along a book. Don't go into a trance and order double shots of Jack Daniels and gulp them down one after the other. Don't try to make a joke out of looking at your watch after you've been caught doing it. Don't keep saying, "What's your name again?" to your date. Don't bring along a briefcase. Don't be an ass.

6. **WHEN YOU GET BACK HOME.** You may well realize that, despite everything, your blind date is the best person you've gone out with in months—something you weren't composed enough to see during the heat of the date itself. Maybe you'd even like to go out on another date. Maybe it could even lead to true you-know-what. Only one thing to do: Sit by the telephone and hope that the feelings were mutual.

## THE SINGLES SCENE

No one likes the singles scene, yet everyone who is not married is in it. We all know that the scene is filled with empty-headed chatter, people asking each other what their signs are, desperate eleventh-hour propositions, and the sound of breaking glass. We all know that the only lasting relationships to come out of such nights on the town are the ones between ourselves and our neuroses.

Nevertheless, when Friday night rolls around, the neurotics are out there flocking together, hoping to stir up a little business, trying to establish a little eye contact.

## Do You Live around Here?

The people in the singles scene are looking for companionship, understanding, and love, to be sure, but first and foremost they are searching for the perfect opening line. Unfortunately, there is no such thing as the perfect opening line; there are merely good ones and bad ones, and the good ones sound rehearsed while the bad ones just sound bad. Neurotics, however, are firm disciples of the opening line. They believe, quite correctly, of course, that without the opener there can be no further discourse. What they don't seem to realize is that even a great opening line in no way guarantees that the ensuing conversation will be any good at all.

In any case, here are a few typically neurotic opening lines:

1. "Do you know anything about ingrown toenails?"

2. "I hate this place, don't you?"

3. "Oh! I'm sorry, I thought you were someone else."

4. "Careful! I've got poison ivy on my arm. See?"

5. "Do you mind if I put my crutches here?"

6. "Vell, vell, vell . . ." (humorous German accent)

7. "Do you know if there's a post office around here anyplace?"

8. "Boy, it's nice to sit down. Do you like to sit down?"

9. "Do you by any chance know what time it is? In China?"

10. "Where did you get them shoes?" (humorous bad grammar)

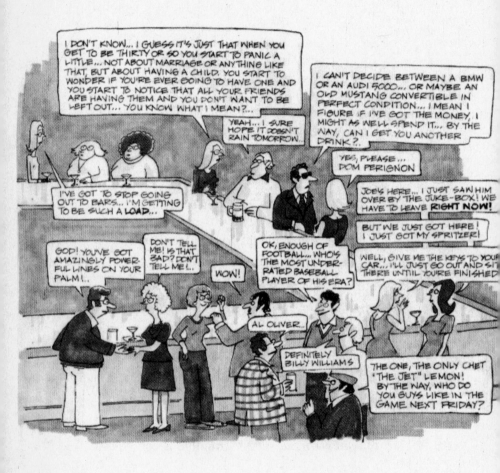

# THOSE THREE LITTLE WORDS

There are times when dating, the singles scene, or even a chance encounter leads to love. At least the neurotic *thinks* it's love. This leads to many joys and problems, of course, but one of the earliest problems is the inability of some neurotics to say, "I love you." It means so much to them to say these words, such a commitment, and, besides, they've been burned so many times before. Frankly, they are tired of saying, "I love you." Why should *they* always have to take the initiative? Why should they once again *lay their whole lives out on the line* just so they can run the risk of hearing the person in question come back with "You do?" or "Don't be ridiculous" or "I've got a train to catch"?

The fact that these neurotics eventually learn not to be the first to say, "I love you" does not prevent them from falling in love (even repeatedly), however. Nor does it prevent them from expressing this love in a thousand other ways. If you hear a partner whom you know to be neurotic utter any of the following, for instance, you'd better start preparing for what lies ahead (or consult the train schedule). If you find yourself saying any of this, you are yet again in over your head.

1. "You can use my car any time you need it."
2. "I really like your family."
3. "Your lip curls up (down) in the nicest way."
4. "Don't you think it would look better if this chair went over there?"
5. "I used your toothbrush."
6. "Sex really doesn't mean *that* much to me."
7. "I haven't felt this relaxed in months."

8. "You can always come to my parents' house for Thanksgiving."

9. "I think the scars give you character."

10. "I hate you."

# THE BIG EVENT

What it all eventually leads to for most of us, whether or not we have found the truer-than-true-love-of-our-lives, is marriage. There are two bits of evidence that suggest the decision to get married is not always a rational one. First, the institution of marriage declares that we are prepared to live in peace and harmony with one person for the rest of our lives. Second, *any* decision that has anything to do with weddings cannot be said to be rational.

Weddings are like the Olympics for neurotics. Weddings give our anxieties the opportunity to gather together in one place, under the twin flags of Love and Etiquette, for a grand display of what years of bitter experience have taught them. As with the Olympics, the original intent of the wedding has gradually been lost in a fog of social and political maneuvering. As with the Olympics, there are certain wedding "events" that capture the attention of the crowd and bring out the best or worst in the participants.

These events in the Wedding Decathlon can be listed as follows:

1. **THE LOW HURDLES.** In this event, the hurdles of parental and peer approval must be cleared. In modern times, the couple usually have been in training for some time and their performances together have been well documented. This still does not prevent the neurotic feeling among the participants that some of the key judges do not approve.

2. **THE STEEPLECHASE.** Once the announcement has been made and the date set, this race begins. A suitable church must be found, and a posh reception site must be secured. This is a tough and even grueling event, especially if a June wedding is planned, because many other contestants are competing for the same prizes. The anxious belief that the setting for the event, rather than the event itself, is the most important thing can cause strife and a loss of concentration here.

3. **THE INVITATIONAL RELAY.** Among the most neurotic of all events. The judges must decide who gets invited to the wedding and who doesn't, and the results almost always cause disappointment and team dissension. Once again, the sideshow nature of this event distracts the couple from the task of Love and sometimes leads to exchanges that are not smooth or orderly. (Look for some reform in this event in future years, especially in light of the infamous Uncle Frank Boycott in Akron, Ohio, in 1980, which almost brought the entire institution of Marriage to its knees when the Ludgen family delegation refused to attend the ceremony until Frank Ludgen—a well-meaning lush—was invited.)

4. **THE MARATHON.** This event tests the legs and the hearts of the participants. It lasts from the day the announcement is made to a day about two weeks before the wedding—a matter of months or, when both participants are extremely neurotic, years. There are peaks and valleys along this marathon course, as well as running through high and low altitudes. Participants say that this is the event that tells them more about themselves than they care to know. The race is very anxiety-producing in its late stages. Most finish it, although some are in such frazzled condition that they barely realize what they are doing along the rest of the way.

5.  **THE VAULT.** An event for the father of the bride. He must exercise agility and legerdemain and grace under fire as the bills start to pour in. The more he has in the vault, the better off he is.

6.  **THE HIGH HURDLES.** The strain is beginning to show as this event rolls around. The hurdles are those of self-doubt and fear, and one slip here can put the whole Decathlon in jeopardy. This is where good coaching becomes imperative. The contestants must be told that the team is more important than the individual, that a similar opportunity may not come up again for years, that the weekend plans of scores of people hang in the balance. If necessary, the dazed participants may be kicked over these key hurdles.

7.  **THE BUTTERFLY.** A few days before the wedding, giant butterflies appear in the stomachs of the major participants and begin to flutter madly. These butterflies feed on small details that suddenly assume enormous proportions. For instance, if the weather forecast calls for a 20 percent chance of rain, the fear is of a torrential tropical downpour that drowns wedding guests in the church parking lot. If a bartender calls in sick, the fear is that the guests will be forced to stand before row upon row of glittering, unopened bottles, muttering nasty oaths against the families of the bride and groom. What if the marriage official turns out to be a long-winded fool? Do we have enough champagne? Where will people park? There is nothing that can make the butterflies go away.

8.  **THE DASH.** This event takes place on the day of the wedding. It is run in a state of high panic, in a wild variety of directions, but ultimately to the same finish line. The Dash is run on a reserve of pure neurotic energy that is so intense it often lights up the bride's face into a radiant flush.

9. **THE TOSS.** When the bride tosses her bouquet, there is one neurotic in the crowd of unmarried females who is convinced that everyone is secretly rooting for her to catch it. She is right. Sometimes the bride will fire the bouquet on a wicked line drive to this woman, but more often an over-enthusiastic thirteen-year-old who knows nothing of lost love and heartache will lunge out and make the grab.

10. **THE CRAWL.** The final event in the Decathlon is meant for the wedding guests. The reception starts out as a super-charged celebration, but, as hour after hour ticks by, it slows to a statelier pace and finally to a crawl. Points are scored during the Crawl for crankiness, the dredging up of dark family secrets, and food and drink spillage, but the only true winners are the bride and groom, who have long since escaped, in a shower of rice, to live happily ever after.

# THE NEUROTIC'S
# HALL OF FAME

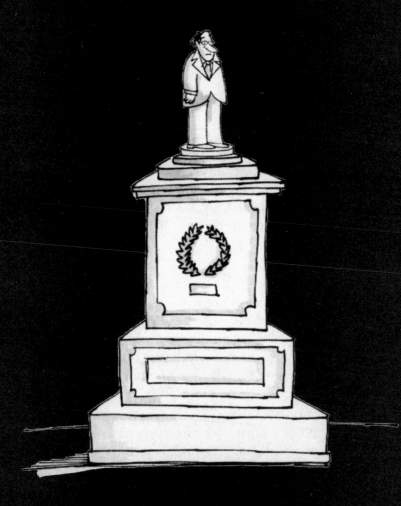

There are neurotics such as you and me and the guy in the back seat of the bus who keeps blowing his nose, and then there are the Great Neurotics. From all walks of life they come, these Great Neurotics, from history and fiction and the entertainment arts they emerge, marching together, out of step, absorbed in their own thoughts and in the way the breeze plays through their hair.

**JOHN ADAMS.** "I have had poverty to struggle with; envy, jealousy and malice of enemies to encounter, no friends, or but few, to assist me; so that I have groped in dark obscurity. . . ." That was Adams at age thirty, not sounding very much like presidential timber and sounding much more like a potential assassin. A neurotic, if able, snob from a New England family steeped in self-abnegation.

**JOHN QUINCY ADAMS.** "I have indulged too much indolence and inactivity of mind, and have not turned my leisure time to good account." A chip off the old Adams block delivering the classic complaint of the driven mind. So in need of approval that he ran for a seat in Congress *after* having served as president.

**MARGIE ALBRIGHT.** The hyperactive heroine of television's *My Little Margie*. The opposite side of the neurotic coin from the brooding Adams clan, she was as jumpy (and as pensive) as a waterbug. Sort of a combination Little Lulu and Little Iodine grown older and come to television, Margie was simply too fast for men like her father, Vern, and her boyfriend, Freddy, to handle. Her great neurotic trait was that although she was in a constant swirl of activity, she never actually *did* anything.

**WOODY ALLEN.** The urban neurotic in the movies and perhaps in real life as well. Neurotic traits: dissatisfaction with being "just a comedian"; constant references to therapy; dresses down for fancy occasions; avoids the Oscars; is purposely not funny during most interviews; throws a blanket of secrecy around all his projects.

**HANS CHRISTIAN ANDERSEN.** Given to wild exhilaration and deep despair throughout his life; often burst into tears at the slightest provocation. Frequently claimed to be working on more profound writing than his children's stories, but never produced anything else. Is said to have stuffed newspapers into his shirt because he was embarrassed by his sunken chest.

**LUDWIG VAN BEETHOVEN.** As he grew older, the composer became a victim of sudden rages, uncontrolled emotions, ungrounded suspicions, and an obsession with money. This last trait was exemplified by his continual haggling over the price of rolls and coffee at Vienna restaurants and his demanding to see the bill before his food had even arrived at the table.

**ALEXANDER GRAHAM BELL.** "I often feel like hiding myself away in a corner out of sight. Whenever I try to say something I stop all conversation." Not a bad reason for inventing the telephone. Bell, who regularly retired at 4 A.M. and had to be rousted out of bed at noon, was known to hide in the attic or lock himself in the bathroom in order to avoid going to parties. Most curiously, he greatly feared having moonlight fall on him as he slept. On nights of the full moon he walked through the house pulling curtains and placing screens to protect the rest of his family from the hideous light.

**THE 1978 BOSTON RED SOX.** The neurotic's Dream Team. Unable to deal with success, the Sox performed one of the great swan dives of modern times. After staking themselves to an extraordinary lead, the talent-laden lineup inexplicably began to bicker and grow sullen. The bats fell silent, the bullpen died, the Yankees advanced. The fans went into an ecstasy of self-denial that was made even sweeter when the Red Sox rallied to force the Yanks into a playoff game—and then lost.

**BENJAMIN BRADDOCK.** The title character in *The Graduate,* Braddock makes a good case for water as a balm for the neurotic soul. During his extended period of inaction and indecision at home, what does he do? He sits on his bed and stares at fish in an aquarium, he lies on a float in the middle of a swimming pool, and at last he dons scuba gear and goes underwater. Trouble ahead.

**CHARLIE BROWN.** The football that is snatched up just as he kicks at it, the kite that is forever tangled in a tree, the baseball team that cannot win, the unattainable red-haired girl—all the problems of a confirmed neurotic. That Charlie Brown is a child probably makes us feel a little better; maybe the problems eventually will go away. But they never do, and Charlie never gets any older or wiser. As for Lucy the Psychiatrist . . .

**JOHN CALVIN.** The father of the doctrine of predestination, which, in turn, might be held responsible for the neurotic's oft-repeated "What's the use?"

**HOLDEN CAULFIELD.** The neurotic adolescent. Surrounded by creeps and phonies, distrustful of anyone over the age of thirty, mortified by the idea of sex, ill at ease in the world. "You can't ever find a place that's nice and peaceful, because there isn't any. You may *think* there is, but once you get there, when you're not looking, somebody'll sneak up and write 'Fuck you' right under your nose. Try it sometime."

**EMILY DICKINSON.** The "Amherst Myth" avoided people to the extent that she ran away whenever the doorbell rang. By age thirty she retreated even when old friends came to visit, instead listening to their voices from her room upstairs. Finally, she spent her last fifteen years as a total recluse. She dressed exclusively in white and in the fashions of her youth until the day she died. She could not wrap packages or address letters, and she was afraid of "prowling boogers." Her doctor was supposed to diagnose her as she walked, fully clothed, by an open doorway.

**FREDERICK EXLEY.** "My stamina was such that most of the time I'd complete no more than three or four sentences run together precisely the way I wanted them, and by then I would be literally too tired to sit up in a chair. Rising . . . I would take the half-dozen steps to the bed . . ." And so on. From Exley's *A Fan's Notes,* a classic novel-memoir of daydreaming and despair in the modern world.

**BOBBY FISCHER.** Chess is the neurotic's ultimate board game, combining an obsessive concern for the near future with an anxious construction of defense mechanisms. Bobby ("Chess is life") Fischer is perhaps the ultimate neurotic chess master. During his epic match in 1972 with Boris Spassky at Reykjavik, Fischer complained that the lighting was too dim, the chess pieces were too small for the squares on the board, the board itself should have been made of wood rather than stone, the orange juice was too warm, the presence of cameras did not allow him to think clearly, and he was a victim of an Icelandic/Communist conspiracy. Astoundingly, the Russians topped all this by having Fischer's chair taken apart after the matches to search for an electronic device with which they thought the winner may have been zapping Spassky's brain.

**SIGMUND FREUD.** But of course. Freud worried that he had a tainted heredity and thought he was doomed to die in 1907 (he made it to 1939). He suffered from a pseudocardiac condition and thought his doctor was keeping the bad news from him. Neurotic jotting (to a friend): "I had all sorts of other good ideas for you during the last few days, but they have all disappeared again. I must wait for the next drive forward, which will bring them back."

**GEORGE IV.** Woke up around 7 A.M. but usually didn't get out of bed until ten hours later. The Crown would breakfast, read every newspaper very thoroughly (a key neurotic trait), transact a bit of business, doze for four or five hours, then get up. At night he'd ring the servants' bell thirty or forty times for such things as asking his valet the time rather than turning to look at a watch that hung beside his bed.

**HETTY GREEN.** Totally concerned with her money, and one of the great misers of all time. Although her fortune (much of which she earned herself) was estimated at over $100 million, she lived in a cold-water flat, wore virtual rags, saved soap slivers, and had her children treated at low-cost medical clinics (perhaps causing her son to lose a leg).

**MARY HARTMAN, MARY HARTMAN.** Perhaps the most wildly realized neurotic character ever to star on a television show. Her actions were usually characterized by guilt, insecurity, or indecision. She was given to nervous twitches, sobbing bouts, free association, and a desperate waving of the hands as she tried to explain something. That a man should drown in a bowl of soup on her kitchen table seemed somehow to be expected.

**MISS HAVISHAM.** The jilted spinster of *Great Expectations,* Miss Havisham chose revenge as the driving force behind her neurosis. She had all the clocks in her house stopped at the moment of her comeuppance while she sat dressed in her yellowed wedding gown in a room with her cobwebbed and rotten wedding cake. Her goal was to raise a girl who would break a young man's heart. She should have been out jogging and loading up on B-group vitamins.

**NATHANIEL HAWTHORNE.** As a young man Hawthorne took to his room and stayed there for years, daydreaming, watching the sunlight move along the wall as the day wore on. "I have made a captive of myself, and put me into a dungeon, and now I can not find the key to let myself out—and if the door were open, I should be almost afraid to come out." Thus, at age thirty-three, was Hawthorne prepared to meet his public.

**HOWARD HUGHES.** Billionaire recluse.

**ALICE JAMES.** The very bright sister of Henry and William remained an invalid for much of her life, although there did not seem to be much physically wrong with her. "Oh woe, woe is me!" she wrote at one point. "I have not only stopped thinning but I am taking unto myself gross fat. All hopes of peace and rest are vanishing—nothing but the dreary snail-like climb up a little way, so as to be able to run down again! And then those doctors tell you that you will die or *recover!* But you *don't* recover. I have been at these alternations since I was nineteen, and I am neither dead nor recovered."

**SAMUEL JOHNSON.** "I hope to put my rooms in order. Disorder I have found one great cause of Idleness." Johnson wrote such notes to himself all his life, but it never seemed to do much good: his rooms remained frightfully messy and he continually fretted over being idle. Dr. Johnson was a textbook case of neurotic tics and habits. He compulsively tapped fence posts with his walking stick as he passed them (and he broke into a nervous sweat if he missed one), he habitually counted his steps from place to place, he grimaced and stretched as he spoke, and he blew out his breath like a whale following a lengthy remark. Johnson was never at ease in this world (he once went as far as to hide in a tree to avoid a visitor). One way he found of coping was to turn to the comparatively straightforward world of mathematics; in times of particular stress he might be found patiently figuring out how many times around the world all the gold in England might be wound if it were pounded down into strips one-fiftieth of an inch thin.

**FRANZ KAFKA.** One of the brighter entries in Kafka's diaries: "Vague hope, vague confidence. An endless, dreary Sunday afternoon, an afternoon swallowing down whole years, its every hour a year. By turns walked despairingly down empty streets and lay quietly on the couch. Occasionally astonished by the leaden, meaningless clouds almost uninterruptedly drifting by. 'You are reserved for a great Monday!' Fine, but Sunday will never end."

**JOHN KEATS.** "I do think better of womankind than to suppose they care whether Mister John Keats five feet high likes them or not." Sure, John.

**ABRAHAM LINCOLN.** Given to dark moods and mysticism. Wrote in 1841: "I am now the most miserable man living. If what I feel were equally distributed to the whole human family, there would not be one cheerful face on earth. Whether I shall ever be better, I cannot tell; I awfully forebode I shall not."

**MARY TODD LINCOLN.** Just what Abe didn't need. She was a bright, well-read woman whose behavior took a rather odd turn once she realized she could never compete with her husband. She threw lavish entertainments in Washington at the height of the Civil War, she berated her husband when he was late to meals, and, more to the point here, she once bought more than three hundred pairs of gloves in a span of four months.

**JAMES MADISON.** As a young man he was victimized by brooding inertia, seizures, paralysis—all of a neurotic nature—and a wish for an early death. "I am too dull and infirm now to look out for any extraordinary things in this world, for I think my sensations for many months have intimated to me not to expect a long or a healthy life. . . ." He lived to be eighty-five.

**COTTON MATHER.** Total self-absorption, total self-analysis, total obsession with sin. When he dressed in the morning he'd consider each part of his body, how it might sin, and how he could prevent it from doing so. He felt an obligation to personally look into any report of sin or scandal within his congregation. He found life with his third wife difficult because she often brought him to the brink of "Enjoyment."

**FLORENCE NIGHTINGALE.** After serving tirelessly on battlefields all over the Empire, Florence Nightingale turned the tables at age forty and became a voluntary invalid. For six years she insisted upon being carried from place to place and for the most part she was content to stay in bed. Following a period of partial recovery, she, at age fifty-two, decided she was dying and requested permission to live as a patient in St. Thomas Hospital until she did so. Since there was nothing particularly wrong with her (fainting spells, extreme weakness), she was dissuaded from her plan. She lived another forty years.

**MARCEL PROUST.** The French novelist spent the last seventeen years of his life in his cork-lined room at 102 boulevard Haussmann, in bed, writing. This neurotic fantasy come to life evolved as Proust, always sickly and nervous, found he simply no longer could stand the sounds and smells of life. Proust feared brain tumors and dizzy spells, he slept fully clothed, even including gloves, and he regularly burned choking amounts of fumigation powder in his room. He also licked the neurotic's problem of how to fit everything on the bedside table: he had three tables within easy reach—one contained books, hot water bottles, and handkerchiefs; the second held a lamp, a watch, pens, spectacles, notebooks, and an inkwell; the third was for his Evian water and lime, coffee, and ritual morning croissant. Naturally, Proust wrote obsessively (and in obsessive detail) about the past.

**LUCY RICARDO.** The neurotic housewife gone berserk, Lucy (of television's *I Love Lucy*) lived in a world of vivid fantasy and utter confusion, her consuming goal being to get her husband to pay attention to her (he was able to do little else). As a true neurotic, Lucy was brilliant in her ability to enlist others (Fred and Ethel Mertz) to help out in her unlikely schemes, and she was gloriously penitent when the schemes, inevitably, backfired. Would it be going too far to say that she was the neurotic conscience of the silent, housebound 1950s?

**JOHANN SCHILLER.** The German writer was unable to work unless he could smell the scent of rotting apples. He kept one in a desk drawer at all times.

**ARTHUR SCHOPENHAUER.** The philosopher posited the neurotic belief that happiness and pleasure are undesirable achievements and that life is a constant struggle to ward off suffering and pain. Personally, he was highly fearful of robbers (he slept with loaded pistols), disease, and poison. His closest companion was his dog.

**DYLAN THOMAS.** "The ordinary moments of walking up village streets, opening doors or letters, speaking good-day to friends or strangers, looking out of windows, making telephone calls, are so inexplicably (to me) dangerous that I am trembling all over before I get out of bed in the morning to meet them." Free-floating anxiety, later drowned in drink.

**DANIEL TOMPKINS.** The vice-president of the United States under Monroe once characterized his life as "toilsome days, sleepless nights, anxious cares, domestic bereavements, impaired constitution, debilitated body, unjust abuse and censure, and accumulated pecuniary embarrassments." And he was only a heart palpitation away from the presidency.

**ANTHONY TROLLOPE.** The English writer constantly fretted about his word production. "According to the circumstances of the time . . . I have allotted myself so many pages a week," he wrote. "The average number has been about 40. It has been placed as low as 20, and has risen to 112. And as a page is an ambiguous term, my page has been made to contain 250 words; and as words, if not watched, will have a tendency to straggle, I have had every word counted as I went." Trollope wrote with a pocket watch placed before him on the table; he strove to write 250 words every 15 minutes.

**FELIX UNGER.** The *Odd Couple* character is perhaps the most widely recognized model of the modern neurotic. The compulsive neatness, the sinus problems and attendant use of an atomizer, the constant near hysteria, and the martyrish, remonstrative "Oscar, *Oscar,* Oscar . . ." were all played for laughs, just as they should have been. Everyone knows a "Felix."

**DUKE OF WELLINGTON.** The duke was known to be so horrified at the idea of being late for an appointment that he sometimes carried six watches.

## ABOUT THE AUTHOR

**CHARLES A. MONAGAN** is the author of several books whose writing has appeared in numerous magazines and newspapers. He lives anxiously in Connecticut.

## ABOUT THE ILLUSTRATOR

**MICK STEVENS**'s illustrations have appeared in *The New Yorker* since 1979 and have been collected in several books. He lives on Martha's Vineyard.